Relapse No More: The Way Out

Guide to Emotional Sobriety and Breaking Self-Destructive Patterns

by Layla Grace

This content is for educational purposes only and is not meant as medical advice or to substitute for treatment by a qualified healthcare provider.

All rights reserved by Grace Revealed LLC.

No part of this book may be reproduced in any manner whatsoever without written permission except in the case of brief quotations embodied in critical articles and reviews.

First Printing, 2024 in the United States of America

979-8-218-33847-3

RELAPSE NO MORE

RELAPSE NO MORE

The Way Out

Guide to Emotional Sobriety & Breaking Self-Destructive Patterns

LAYLA GRACE

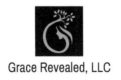

Grace Revealed, LLC

CONTENTS

Dedication	ix
Disclaimer	2
Introduction	4
1 Understanding The Problem	6
2 Recognizing Patterns	15
3 Preparing for Transformation	25
4 Freedom Protocol	34
5 Handling Setbacks	57
6 Balancing Boundaries	68
7 Emotional Sobriety	88
8 Get Well, Be Well, Stay Well	95
Conclusion	118
Grace Revealed LLC	122
Stay In Touch	123

Acknowledgements 125
About The Author 126

Dedication

This book is to my fellow recovering addicts who have struggled to put down food, sex, drugs, alcohol, a negative person, a toxic family member or anything in-between that is taking away and not adding to your peace of mind.

This book is to anyone struggling with emotional pain who is looking for a pathway to peace.

This book is for you, my friend. This book is to encourage you and help you keep going. You will break those negative patterns and adopt some new ones, once and for all! Keep going. Do not give up.

"Life begins at the end of your comfort zone."

~Neal Donald Walsch

Relapse No More

The Way Out

*Guide to Emotional Sobriety and
Breaking Self-Destructive Patterns*

By Layla Grace

Disclaimer

In the chapters to come you are going to hear about burnout, what my life was like before, and what it's like after burnout. You will discover the path that leads to rewiring the brain from hurting to healing. You will learn how to help others do the same. We are going to talk about feelings; what they tell us and what to do with them. You will be empowered to let go and overcome "trying to control" the universe. We are going to learn; about connecting with others, finding a healing environment where change is possible, and how to go from chaos to order in our lives. We are also going to discuss restoration. *Relapse No More* is about being able to recognize when we are tempted to self-harm and have a process to take care of ourselves that will open the doors to new opportunities of transformation and change. Finally, we will talk about how to enjoy life after we break negative self-destructive patterns.

For some people it might feel weird and uncomfortable to come out of dysfunction and into a place of peace. I assure you, when you are surrounded by the right, life-giving people, you will know peace deep down. You will know a peace of mind that cannot be taken away from you, a new freedom and a new happiness.

A Challenge

A small challenge to you for when you're really serious about seeing transformation and change inside yourself. Be gentle with yourself, take it one day at a time, or maybe 1 hour at a time, and do not give up. I promise, when you put the work into yourself, the reward will be beyond your imagination. Keep going.

Note: Being emotionally overwhelmed is real. There is help. If you're currently experiencing overwhelming emotional pain and want it healed, visit **www.GraceRevealedllc.com/book** and schedule an appointment to talk. Check out the Freedom Protocol that will help hijack your brain for freedom from the pain and set you on the path to well-being. We look forward to being part of your healing journey!

Introduction

I will never forget that one Friday night. I was at the grocery store and it was well after dinner time. Late on a Friday night and here I was in the prepared food section desperately hanging on to my small shopping cart. White-knuckling. I knew I was getting ready for a binge because I could not stop the emotional pain I was in. What was the trigger? I have no idea. All I knew was, I wanted the emotional pain to stop, and numbing myself with food was the only, quickest way I knew that might still be legal.

That is addiction. Addiction is when we want to stop ourselves and cannot. Addiction is a negative self-destructive pattern that is set off by a trigger and keeps going until the pain is stopped, by triggering the pleasure center in the brain. It is an addiction because if we could stop ourselves we would have done it by now. If that's you, I invite you to come all the way in, sit all the way down and hear the steps that will help set you free.

Food is one of the most cunning, baffling and powerful addictions I've ever seen. Being addicted to flour and sugar has often been minimized, but I assure you, it is one of the most challenging "process addictions" to overcome - aside from having an intimacy disorder. For I know, none other addictions, that are more difficult to overcome than food and intimacy because we need Food and Connection to survive life.

My story is filled with much hope and healing from the tremendous pain and suffering I've endured at the hand of my abusive father, borderline personality mother, my childhood friend's brother who took advantage of me and countless others I let treat me like garbage.

That night, I cried out to God and asked for help and found a solution that led me down a path, to heal mentally, physically, spiritually and emotionally. I am now years into my right-sized body. I discovered a path that breaks patterns of self-harm and creates new patterns in the brain, for self-care that leads to life. It works, if you work it. Are you ready to try something different?

When you're ready and want change, reading this book gives you the way out that will work for you when you apply the tools and lessons spelled out for you in the pages ahead. If you don't want change, you won't change. To the brave, willing and courageous readers… Take what you like, and leave the rest.

Let's dive in!

CHAPTER 1

Understanding The Problem

Recognition. What is the problem?

Welcome to the beginning. What's the problem? If we don't know what the problem is then why would we need a solution? Each one of us will have to answer this question for ourselves: What is the negative pattern that you are up against, right now? When it feels like there are several obstacles in your way, please just focus on one primarily for now. Pick the one negative behavior that *if you could stop this today*, it would make your life a whole life a lot better. What is that one area? Let's focus clearly on that, and we can address the others later.

Defining Addiction

For the purpose of this book, we want to start with an understanding that individuals do not wake up one day and think "I want to be an addict". Addiction is not a choice. Addiction is when an individual gets stuck in a cycle and the ability to stop is lost. It is a relapsing disorder characterized by compulsive use (or behavior) despite negative consequences. Addiction is a complex and multifaceted condition that affects individuals from all walks of life.

Addiction can manifest in various forms. Right? Addictions such as substance abuse, behavioral addictions and process addictions. For Example: emotional eating, over-consumption, sexual compulsion, drug use, alcohol abuse, pornography, self-mutilation, and anything that you can picture as compulsive and difficult to stop with will-power alone.

Addiction and self-sabotage are complex. They have intricate issues that affect individuals differently. Throughout this text, I will share with you my experience, strength and hope around overcoming and breaking free of tangled issues. This book is to help you overcome self-destructive patterns and live with emotional sobriety and a lasting sound mind.

That said, I encourage you to take what you like and leave the rest. The most important part is to put into practice the things that resonate with you, your journey and the current phase and process of where you are today, on the path of healing.

Understanding addiction or self-destructive patterns must start with identifying the problem; the fruit, what is the negative thing that we need to change? If you have a flat tire on your car you cannot just change *any* tire, you have to change only the tire that is flat! There's the old adage that says... "if it's not broken, don't fix it" and we are applying that here, today. If it **is** broken we want a solution! We have to identify **what is broken** first. Then we will unravel the underlying causes behind it, so that we can walk-out the solution.

The Cycle of Addiction

As we understand addiction, it happens in cycles. Noticeable patterns have been studied and defined in stages. There are four stages typical with Addiction and Relapse: initiation, escalation, maintenance, and relapse.

Initiation: This stage marks the beginning of the addiction cycle. It often involves the initial exposure to a substance or behavior that provides pleasure or relief. At this stage, individuals may experiment with drugs, alcohol, or engage in addictive behaviors, finding temporary enjoyment or relief from stress or emotional pain.

Escalation: In the escalation stage, the frequency and intensity of substance use or addictive behaviors increase. Tolerance develops, meaning that individuals require larger amounts or more frequent engagement to achieve the same desired effect.

This stage is characterized by a loss of control, as individuals find it increasingly difficult to moderate or *stop* their addictive self-harming behaviors.

Maintenance: During the maintenance stage, addiction becomes deeply ingrained in an individual's life. The pursuit of the addictive substance or behavior becomes a central focus, often at the expense of other important aspects of life, such as relationships, work, or personal well-being. Individuals may experience physical and psychological dependence, experiencing withdrawal symptoms when attempting to quit or reduce their addictive behaviors. Maintenance is when we practice the same ritual or pattern over and over that creates grooves into the reward center of the brain to start and maintain the pattern.

Relapse: Relapse refers to a return to addictive behaviors after a period of abstinence or attempts at recovery. It is a common occurrence in the cycle of addiction and can be triggered by various factors, such as stress, emotional turmoil, or exposure to cues associated with the addictive substance or behavior. Relapse does not signify failure but rather highlights the challenges of breaking free from addiction. It requires help outside of the person struggling to be free.

Defining Relapse

Relapse is a common challenge faced by individuals on the path to recovery. It is important to recognize that relapse is not a single event but rather a process that unfolds in stages. By understanding these stages, individuals can develop strategies to prevent and manage relapse effectively.

Emotional Relapse: The first stage of relapse is often characterized by emotional and mental patterns that set the stage for future relapse. During this stage, individuals may experience increased stress, anxiety, or emotional turmoil. They may neglect self-care, isolate themselves, or engage in negative thinking patterns. It is crucial to recognize and address these emotional triggers to prevent further progression towards relapse.

Mental Relapse: In the second stage, mental relapse, individuals experience a tug-of-war between the desire to use substances or engage in addictive behaviors and the commitment to recovery. Conflicting thoughts and cravings emerge, with part of the mind longing for the addictive behavior while another part recognizes the negative consequences. Urges and fantasies about using become more frequent, and individuals may start romanticizing past substance use or addictive behaviors.

Physical Relapse: The final stage of relapse is physical relapse, where individuals actually engage in addictive behavior or substance use. This stage is often the culmination of the preceding emotional and mental relapse stages. It is important to note that physical relapse does not occur suddenly but is the result of a process that can be interrupted at any stage. Recognizing the stages of relapse empowers individuals to intervene early and prevent a full-blown relapse. By addressing emotional triggers, developing healthy coping mechanisms, seeking support, and implementing relapse prevention strategies, individuals can navigate the challenges of recovery more effectively. It is crucial to remember that relapse does not signify failure but rather an opportunity for growth and learning on the journey towards sustained recovery.

Okay, we don't need another book on what addiction is. Look at the 12 Steps of AA (Alcoholics Anonymous) or visit your local bookstore. This book is about the Way Out! When you *know* you want to **stop** a pattern and cannot, this book gives you a new way to practice life by breaking those addictive patterns and living free of the constant loop of self-sabotage. Let's prepare to dig in!

Currently Struggling

Much compassion to you if you are currently struggling with chronic relapse and the pain of reaping the consequences of not being able to stop that addictive self-destructive pattern. Please keep going. Do not give up. As long as you are breathing, there is hope!

Try grabbing a journal or a pen and paper to keep track of where you're at on this journey and what tools in this book you can start to implement and practice today. This is where change starts to happen. By now, your primary area of help should be identified and kept in mind as we transition forward in the book. Let's look at it from the perspective of a renovation building project.

The Transformation Process

Like any good renovation project in construction, going back to the foundation is important. When you are going through this process, you may feel like your life is one big construction site and that is perfectly okay for now. Demolition. Overhaul. Reconstruction. Celebration.

Let's close down this chapter with a Construction site *visual*:

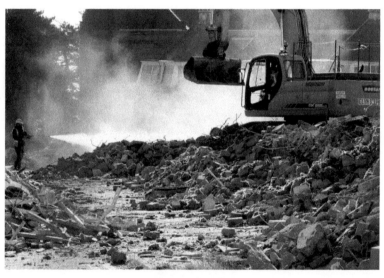

Construction Site
https://pixabay.com/photos/digger-excavator-demolition-6955736/

Photo 1.0

Question: What state of construction is your life in?

The best type of transformational change is one that happens down at the very foundation. One of the best phrases that you could hear on a construction site is "safety first". We need to feel safe when we are going to change. I give you permission to unravel and let the transformation process take place. The most lasting change from the inside-out develops with a *process* and not just a one-time experience. The best change is gradual. Little by little.

Final Consideration

So, I ask you to begin to loosen up your grip of control on what you think your life *should* look like and let it unravel before you. Building from the bottom makes the best foundation and that means that we will need the roots to be dug up and a new Foundation to be put in place. This will add the best structure for us to build on, going forward.

Let's begin by identifying the one thing that you are struggling with the most. Write it down and visualize what stage of construction you are in, to prepare for a healing transformation from the things that have tried to trip you up! Block away the other distractions or struggles that might be tempting you to steal your focus and we will start making progress.

Chapter 1 Summary:

In this chapter we defined addiction and reviewed the cycle of addiction to better understand relapse. We considered many forms of negative behavior that have become challenging to break with willpower alone. We looked at understanding relapse and saw that it is tricky, complex and a form of bondage when we lose the ability to choose a better healthier choice. We understand that we cannot change, even when we want to, without help. The nature of addiction. We also heard there is a way out.

See you in the next chapter!

CHAPTER 2

Recognizing Patterns

A Starting Point

Awareness. We have to recognize our own patterns of self-destructive Behavior so that we can break the mold. I hate to keep focusing on "the problem" but it is important to have recognition of what our own personal patterns look like so that we can understand how we are going to break those particular patterns! These chronic cycles take life from us. They are unable to add life to us! See the difference? One behavior brings value and enhances our lives, the other degrades and is never satisfied.

Before Recovery

I thought I had it "all together" on the outside. Had a good job, bought a house, loved my car and was actively serving in almost every area of "the church" I could… I was striving for "ada-girls" from bosses, pastors and anyone who would give me praise for "doing" whatever I was "doing" for a sense of approval. I would go to great lengths for YOU to "APPROVE" of me.

I suppose growing up, being the 3rd of 9 children in a household full of pain wouldn't have anything to do with it, would it? Where my dad was working A Lot and Emotionally UNAVAILABLE when he was home? What about a mom who was consistently scheming up drama to infuriate my dad with, while blaming it on "the children"? I eventually learned that my dad was secretly hiding his homosexual lifestyle and my mom was practicing the dark art of witchcraft that was not in alignment with God's light or love - at all.

As early as 7 years old, I was trained to jump in dumpsters for food, clothing and anything else I could find that would be better than the hand-me-downs from my older sisters. At age 13, my dad taught me to drive the family van so I could be ready to cart my siblings around, as needed.

One of my most painful memories was when my mom would gather us for a "Family Meeting" to announce that ANOTHER sibling was ON-The-Way! It happened approximately every-other year, and a sick feeling of rejection washed over me - EVERY time, because They wanted A Boy! And I was wrong, unacceptable and unwanted. At this "announcement" I just wanted to run away and escape the pain of rejection. Eventually, in the kitchen, I stumbled upon a sugary substance in the cupboard that took-the-edge-off, quickly. I ate and ate that stuff until it made me sick. Man! Did it make me feel good though!

Common Self-Destructive Patterns

Here they are: The "not good enough" lie, isolation, denial and the "victim" mentality. We will look a little deeper at each one, in this chapter. When I was in my darkest hour, I could barely see the patterns that were defiling my life. As I admitted that I needed help and couldn't break the patterns on my own, awareness started to flow in. Awareness of my self-harm problem (couldn't stop hurting myself) was the first place. Admitting that I needed help was second. This awareness brought light into the dark places of my mind.

The Not Good Enough (lie)

One common self-destructive pattern is negative self-talk. "I'm not good enough, I'm not smart enough, I'm not rich enough, I'm not pretty enough or handsome enough". Negative patterns of thought become easy to "believe" when we have had the thought reinforced by a memory of other people treating us poorly.

Often we need a right-sized perspective of ourselves to keep humble. We do NOT need a voice in our heads to belittle us or say we are not enough. Let me be the voice of truth in your mind today. You are enough. Smart enough. Worthy. You are worthy enough *to be still long enough* to get clear about healing from self-sabotaging choices.

Maybe I never felt "Good Enough", because I repeatedly heard "You were supposed to be a boy" and "Don't tell anyone" about the chronic abuse and depravity our eventual family of 11 people was experiencing, day in and day out. Parents who said one thing and did something else. Who created chaos at every turn, instead of living in the light. All I knew is: THERE had to be MORE to Life than this insanity! Deep down, I knew there was a bigger Plan for me, although I had little understanding of HOW to grasp God's will for my life. I kept trudging forward at attempts to fill the voids of self-worth and value going it alone and making several attempts to "figure it out" by myself. Please hear the Caution Sign to the "independent spirits" who like to "go it alone". Being alone too long is dangerous territory.

Here is another subtle one... Isolation.

Isolation

Isolation is another self-destructive pattern. It sounds like... "I have to figure it out. If I don't do it, who will?" "Let me just research this some more. I don't want to be a bother." "No one cares what's going on with me." These beliefs and negative self-talk subtly "justifies" a hurting person to isolate and cut themselves off from connection. It is a trap.

Let me tell you: isolation equals death. How about self-sabotage? When you have an opportunity to add value to yourself, do it! Don't *cut yourself off* from hanging out with people, going to worship or pray, and instead binge on Netflix and ignore the life that you've been given.

Then, there is impulsive behavior, like: hooking up with someone that you don't even know, binging into a state of oblivion, eating so much you become food drunk, or texting someone even when you know they don't really even care about you.

Denial

Denial is another one. Denial is tricky. Sometimes, we don't even know that we are in a place of denial. The point is that these patterns can manifest in different aspects of our lives such as: relationships, work, and our own personal well-being. Stay alert and welcome reflections from others to offer you an appropriate view of yourself. The voice of pride gets tricky when it comes to denial.

Secretly Powerless

WE are truly only "as sick as our secrets" and only the truth will set us free.

Before recovery, my lowest part was realizing that I had become completely POWERLESS over Food and my addiction to people-please was running me into the ground. I was experiencing burnout and my organs had begun shutting down. My quality of the life was plummeting. I found myself in less than appropriate relations with men and saw myself as a bag of garbage on the side of the road, waiting to be tossed aside. Worthless. Of no value. Like the dumpsters I jumped in, throughout my childhood. I felt like garbage. I would scrounge for scraps of love and eat junk food to quiet my aching pain of rejection and anxiety that raged in my mind. I did not know how to properly connect with other human beings, especially that of the opposite sex.

Being hospitalized for my heart pausing several times a day, bed-ridden with my organs shutting down. I had become addicted to excitement (from work deadlines and people pleasing) and my adrenal glands had almost depleted of adrenaline. It was no longer a game of "What could I get away with?" I couldn't get out of bed for 3 months, 6 months, turned into 18 months of chronic fatigue and hope diminishing - for life to go on. Where the heck would I start to find my way to health and well-being? I was truly lost. At my wits end. The lights were about to go out.

During that season, I was chronically *blaming* others for the *results* in my life that came from my own decisions. Most of us have heard, by now, that we reap what we sow, right? That is directly from the Good Book.

I remember a time when I was constantly pointing fingers and blaming other people for my bad choices. I didn't even realize I was doing it, unfortunately. Then, I would get frustrated when friendships would fizzle because they were sick of me blaming *them* for the results of **my** bad choices. I was a product of my dysfunctional family and I had a bad case of the "victim mentality".

Victim Mentality

The victim mentality is a mental trap that keeps adults stuck in a blaming storm. When held accountable for our own choices, the internal finger pointing raises its ugly head! It is not fun to take responsibility for poor choices. Especially the ones that poorly affected someone else too! Ugh. Not fun. While exploring more about that victim mentality, I discovered that it did indeed come from once being a victim. This is an important understanding to let sink in..

Today, I am an adult who can take responsibility for my own choices. Although, I remember seeing a wake of destruction to quality relationships (or what could have been quality relationships) because I kept blaming others for my own bad decisions. It was really sad when I look back on it today.

As I started implementing changes to take radical responsibility for my choices the dynamics in my close relationships really started to improve. The people around me who were sick of me blaming others faded away because they *gave up,* and didn't want to give me another chance. Other people stuck around long enough (with grace) to let me change and begin the process of taking responsibility for my choices one day at a time. One moment at a time and one *new* and better decision at a time.

Here's another example: Look at my body! I am what I eat. I cannot blame anyone else for that. I had to start to make small changes one bite at a time. As I started to make better choices with my food, the change was only a matter of time when people started to notice: 15 lbs. down, then 20 lbs., then 30 lbs., then 60 lbs. Change is not easy but it is good. I discovered when I sowed into LIFE, I was reaping a better LIFE.

Honesty and Integrity

I share these examples to emphasize that these are universal principles that are applicable to anyone who is capable of practicing honesty and integrity. When you want a place to start, start exercising honesty and integrity around the one area that you want complete, total healing and transformation in.

The inevitable truth shows; in our bodies, mind, will and emotions. Negative consequences of self-destructive patterns on a person's life get worse, more dangerous, more destructive on a person's mind, physical body, and emotional stability the longer they stay in those patterns. Not to mention their spiritual well-being or health.

In those days, when I was harming myself, I was putting strain on relationships. I was putting strain on my career, and I was putting strain on my own personal growth. We cannot walk toward change (for the better) and away from change at the same time.

Therefore, I encourage you to engage in some self-reflection and develop awareness of your own self-destructive patterns.

The opposite of self-destruction is self-worth and self-care. Not selfishness.

Consider this:

What is one thing that you could change today that would bring you more peace of mind? What is one thing you could let go of? I want you to get really clear on what you are trying to accomplish. What is the one thing that this book can help you change for good?

Please try not to judge yourself as right or wrong, just *observe* with self-compassion. During this process, see where there is some negative cycle or pattern in your life. Then, notice that if you rid yourself of *it*, that would add value to your life.

Chapter 2 Summary

In this chapter we talked about recognizing self-destructive patterns and choosing awareness. I shared some personal examples and the negative effects that compulsive self-destructive patterns had on my life and can have on a person's life. You've also been challenged to do some self-awareness with a non-judgmental observation to identify one area that you'd like to see change as you continue reading this book. Stay alert and I will see you in the next chapter!

CHAPTER 3

Preparing for Transformation

The Ground has been cleared

Now we are getting into the good stuff. Preparing for the transformation to take place. This is the way out! We are going to look at *strategies* for breaking negative, self-destructive patterns in our lives. We are going to talk about different approaches and a step-by-step guide to help you overcome the challenges and stay motivated when things get challenging.

A baseline for healing is being willing to *feel* your feelings. Oh yay! Feelings. Yes, we must be able to feel if we are going to heal.

What if I can't feel my feelings you ask? In that case, we just start with the *core* feelings: glad, sad, hurt, angry, lonely, afraid, guilt, and shame. Those are the basic and core emotions that

I'm going to ask you to identify and check-in with yourself on a daily basis. The opposite of "checking out" is **checking-in** with ourselves. Stop and ask yourself "How am I doing? ... Really".

Please don't forget a pen and paper or a journal as we dive into this chapter. This is the meat of the book and road map for successful breakthroughs. This life-transforming tool activates when you put it into practice and can change your mind, body and relationships for the better! How do you *feel* about that?

While we are talking about feelings, I want to remind you that emotions are just simply a sign of what's going on inside of us. When negative patterns that are "on loop" in our brains try to betray us, we have to be able to *hear* what is *really* behind the feelings.

Our bodies give us clues and signals of what is going on in our minds. If our mind is sick, our bodies reflect that. When our integrity has been jeopardized, the quickest way to relief is often through an apology and raw honesty.

Key Ingredients for Lasting Change

There are three key factors that will help in this transformation process.

1) Willingness
2) Desire for Change
3) Courage to try something we've never tried before.

Without these three ingredients transformation is nearly impossible. I cannot help you change if you do not want to, no one can. You must have a desire to stop the negative cycle, need willingness and courage to try something new. These tools are no good if we are unwilling to try them.

Without courage to try something new, you will always remain stuck in the old self-destructive pattern. So to my courageous and willing soldiers who want change let's get ready to dig in deeper! Overhaul the old and build the new, brick by brick.

About that...

There was a time when I couldn't feel my feelings because I was too quick to numb them! We numb feelings because they are painful! It is hard to feel when we are numbing, at the same time. Literally, our brains can only do *one* thing at a time. We cannot numb our feelings and attempt to *feel* our feelings at the same time.

On the contrary, when you feel the temptation to numb the feelings there is power in the pause: waiting for a split second, maybe 30 seconds or a minute, or maybe even sleeping on a decision instead of making a knee-jerk reaction. This gives way to possibility for change.

Often, our brains are trained to react, not respond with a wise mind, especially in pain. Therefore, when you pause, you can pay attention to what your feelings are telling you *deep down* before responding to any given situation. This power-pause gives way to ending a life filled with assumptions, and gives way to wonder and curiosity.

I assure you, life is beautiful when you eliminate (or quiet) assumptions in your mind. Replace your assumptions with accurate information. Really "find out" what is behind someone's motive or desire to achieve an outcome.

There are a range of strategies that are very practical at helping individuals break self-destructive patterns. Some examples include: self-reflection, goal setting, positive affirmations, and behavior replacement techniques. There are benefits to each of these strategies.

Each of these strategies contribute to personal growth and Recovery but this book is designed to help stop the relapse cycle once and for all. This tool, I am about to show you, gives hope, not to return to negative self-sabotaging behaviors. So let's look at a few practical strategies, in the next chapter, for breaking the old patterns and finding the new pattern that leads to life.

Bonus Material

By now you should have received the bookmark with some Journal questions on it. Please use them! or visit www.Grace-RevealedLLC.com to order your own copy of the One Day At A Time journal and download our FREE Journal Questions.

These are tools to improve your life, not just in your mind and your emotions, but practically and realistically in your most important relationships and in your spirit.

Self-reflection is a powerful tool when it is done on a very regular and consistent basis. It's important to put yourself first on this journey. I give you permission to take care of yourself first before another plant, pet, or another person. When you are not well, you cannot give to others from a place of abundance.

Self-reflection is a wonderful way to check-in with ourselves and answer how we are doing physically, emotionally, mentally and spiritually. Some of us may need to see a therapist to get a mental health check-up. Or check-in? Some of us may need to see a doctor, a dentist, specialist or get ourselves to a beauty salon to take care of our physical needs. Some of us might need a back massage. Whatever you choose, really check-in with yourself first and ask yourself how you are doing on a scale from 1 to 10, in each area.

Keep it Simple

For me, the strategy of goal setting never worked. The one goal in this book is to *stop* the negative pattern and start a more positive and life-giving pattern. We stop the pattern in our minds first, so we can experience outward change after.

Start by simply putting it together one day at a time. That can lead into one week, and then one year. The process of freedom can be gradually increasing in value.

Valuing self-care, self-worth, and self-compassion are how positive changes are built. Brick by brick. The only goal here is to be well. Do you want to be well?

Seriously, it's one of the most important questions you can answer on a day-to-day basis. Do I want to be well?

I'll never forget the time when I made a clear-cut decision that I wanted to be well, no matter what. I made the decision that well-being was my full-time job. God used little circumstances in my life to help bring healing when I was willing and courageous enough to try.

When you decide that you want to be well, there is an unlimited amount of resources available to help you be well, get well, stay well!

Some examples I remember are hugs that came from my dear friends, interactions with five and seven-year-old children, eye contact sitting in 12-step recovery rooms where people just "got me" and understood where I was coming from.

I remember being able to sit *with* my feelings and understand that "this too shall pass", instead of trying to continue to numb the pain. I was able to listen to the pain and let the pain be a teacher. To hear the lesson from the pain that my own body, mind and spirit were trying to help me learn. I cried and let things out, so I could be well. It was amazing what the God of the Universe unraveled for my healing to take place during this season of demolition and reconstruction.

Picture yourself in this unraveling process. I promise you that healing is yours if you stay willing and courageous to do things that you've never done before. So that you can experience a deeper level of healing that you've never experienced before. It is beyond imagination.

Yes, I do have a bad day from time to time and I do get discouraged occasionally on this path to well-being. But today I have systems and processes set in place so that I never go back to the level of depravity of self-harm that I once did. Our brains are magnificent things and they like to find the shortest, easiest and most convenient way to be comfortable. However, today I choose courage over comfort. I choose belonging over fitting in.

On your journey, I encourage you to choose courage over comfort when things are inconvenient or difficult. Choose belonging by being comfortable in your own skin with who you are and the boundaries you've set for yourself. Don't be who people want you to be. Be who YOU want you to be.

Change is not easy, but it is worth it. So, please do not give up on yourself or give up on others that you want to see change. Change requires a great deal of endurance and effort, but it is worth every ounce of time, effort, and energy that you put into being well. When you get rigorously honest with yourself and another human being, the inner transformation will surpass your imagination.

Chapter 3 Summary:

Change is yours if you are willing to go after it, let go of your painful life as you once knew it, and get ready to embrace a new way of living. Stay committed to the work of well-being and you will change. You mind first, then your will and emotions. As emotional pain lifts off of you, physical pain and the burden of shame will also lift. Watch as you become lighter emotionally and physically when you stay-the-course. Look forward, not backward. Find solutions, not problems.

CHAPTER 4

Freedom Protocol

Your Personal Freedom Protocol

So, let's get into the last strategy for breaking self-destructive patterns and it is called the behavior replacement technique or Freedom Protocol as we call it, at Grace Revealed LLC. There is a *process* to it. I need you to lean hard on your courage, stay focused and determined to be well, as we put together your step-by-step guide to implement this strategy in your life. Are you ready? Let's do it! It's less painful than you might think.

Getting Started

Now this is going to require some blank paper and a writing utensil, preferably a marker if you have one. When you want a buddy or someone to help you with this, sign up for your own personal Freedom Protocol on GraceRevealedLLC.com website! We will set aside an hour of time to meet with you, and overcome one area at a time. This is *your* time to break one area of self-destructive and self-sabotaging patterns and live free from its hold on you.

This will help you have clearly defined steps to break those patterns once and for all. This process will add value by giving you a game plan to stop the relapse cycle. You will begin to experience a fulfilling life for yourself when you are dedicated to not giving up!

When you have a clean sheet of paper, poster board or whatever you have around (and a marker), let's get started.

Step 1: We are going to start by drawing an arch like you see in Figure 1.0.

Draw the arch from left to right.

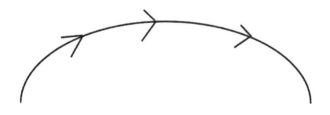

Figure 1.0
Freedom Protocol by Grace Revealed, LLC

NOTE: At this point in the process, be thinking about the *ritual* or process that your *own* brain has taken your body through (at the very point) when you have been triggered by something unexpectedly.

A trigger is something that causes you to enter a particular pattern of thoughts, which leads you to a negative behavior that is harmful or not desirable. This takes us to step two in the drawing process. Keep it simple.

Step 2: Add the word "Trigger" on the left and "Result" on the right. See Figure 1.1

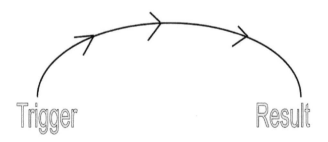

Figure 1.1
Freedom Protocol by Grace Revealed, LLC

As we prepare for the next step in the sequence, simply put something down on the **Right** side of the page that will identify the negative Result that happens when you are triggered. This result happens, even when we don't necessarily want it to. It happens when we are weak or cannot say NO to ourselves. It happens especially on a bad day, leading us to self-sabotage. It happens when we are over-tired and emotionally overwhelmed. Been there! Now, we need to look at what happens in our minds, on the way there. This is called the "ritual".

We are going to start to recognize our own ritual, so that we can identify HOW to break the pattern. Our "ritual" is a pattern of thoughts or behavior that justifies us acting on the negative impulse. See the example below as you begin to fill out your own. Read through the example in Figure 1.2 as you begin to identify your own patterns. No shame here. Just staying aware of the patterns in our minds.

Freedom Protocol - EXAMPLE

Let's use FOOD as an example:

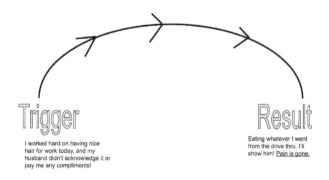

Figure 1.2
Freedom Protocol by Grace Revealed, LLC

Step 4

Recognize the Ritual. What happens in the brain to "justify" acting out (the result) or for some of us, it is "acting-in" (avoiding or not acting) a particular behavior. See Figure 1.3 to draw lines along the way from left to right. Some people may have 3-5 elements in their ritual. We are showing only 3 for our compulsive eating example below.

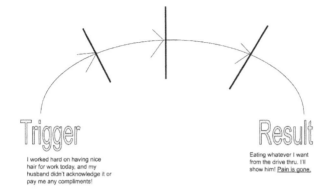

Figure 1.3
Freedom Protocol by Grace Revealed, LLC

Progression. Watch the progression unfold with a Thought, a Justification, and a Rationalization. Sometimes, our brains tell us lies! Be aware.

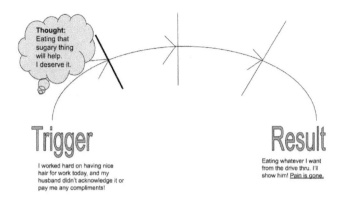

Figure 1.4
Freedom Protocol by Grace Revealed, LLC

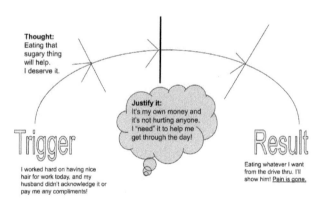

Figure 1.5
Freedom Protocol by Grace Revealed, LLC

Tip: Pay attention to your own "ritual" (brain sequence) next time you are triggered by something. Awareness of our patterns creates the opportunity for change and lessens the impulse to act out.

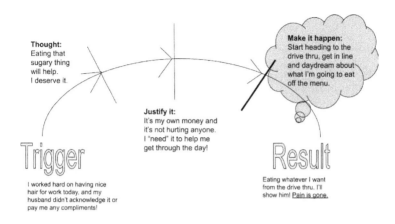

Figure 1.6
Freedom Protocol by Grace Revealed, LLC

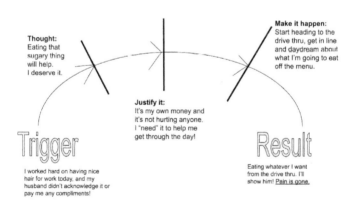

Figure 1.7
Freedom Protocol by Grace Revealed, LLC

That is the self-harm cycle!

Alright. Well done! you made it through the first part in the process. Did you see it happen? Let's talk about what happened:

The trigger.

Let me tell you! it's never about *what* the trigger is. It is **not** about when we get triggered per se.. The only thing to know here is that triggers happen. Trying to control your triggers is an absolute waste of time. They are *triggers* because we don't know what the trigger is or when it will hit us but we DO know that triggers will happen.

A trigger can be anything from a song on the radio to a smell that passes our nose. It could be a noise coming from someone else, or simply a touch from someone without notice. It could be the sound of a zipper.

We never know what the triggers are going to be. For those of us who have tried to stop relapse before, we know that the trigger sets off the path to the "acting out" or the compulsive behavior. That behavior is addictive and self-destructive in nature.

These visuals are to give you an understanding of what happens in the brain that leads us to self-harm. I've watched too many clients attempt to minimize and "control" triggers and fail. What we are doing now is the work needed to develop a process for when you are triggered.

The ritual.

This is when a Thought enters into the picture. Right? Look at the example again. Thought: "Why didn't he acknowledge that my hair looks nice or pay me any compliments?", "I know what can quiet this pain, eating that *sugary* thing will help me. I *deserve* it."

Note: *Everyone's ritual is personal to them. The goal is to identify what yours looks like or sounds like, during this phase.*

Next, the brain goes into *justifying* the compulsive behavior. Sounds like: "It is my own money and it's not hurting anyone." and "I need it to help me get through the day!"

Then, we go out to make it happen! We start heading to the drive-thru, get in line, and start daydreaming about what we are going to order off the menu. We fantasize and are convinced it will end the pain, whether we realize it or not. Indulging in fantasies can be dangerous. We lose focus and stability at this point in the ritual. Our grip on reality seems to fade.

The acting-out.

Or for some, acting-in. This is when the rubber hits the road. The deed is done. We have acted out the compulsion, fantasy or "pleasure" that we talked ourselves into. What you do not see on this graphic is the end result of our actions. Let's play it "all the way through".

The person in our example is Triggered by the fact that their partner didn't pay them a compliment after their attempts at a good hair day! They, then, feel emotionally triggered and a Thought enters their mind to "eat something from the drive-thru" (immediately if possible), instead of having healthy communication.

Next, they justify the purchase and tell themselves lies to "feel better" about doing something they know they will have to pay for later with their health! Lastly, they get in line to "Make It Happen". After they get in line, order whatever they want to comfort eat (numb the pain), they have a full belly and temporarily the emotional pain ends (is numbed).

She was feeling confident and pretty until she didn't get the feedback she wanted. Now that she's eaten to numb the pain, shame comes sneaking around the corner of her mind. Then, the guilt from once again eating that stuff that is making her feel miserable, and packing on the pounds!

Nothing healthy came from numbing the pain (emotionally eating), it was just a temporary escape. Can you see that? Does that example resonate? Okay, that is just completing the full circle on the *problem*. I assure you, it gets better from here!

It Gets Better

Here is where it gets good! This is where breaking the pattern happens. Let's take another look at the graphic and keep our writing utensil handy! We are going to break this *thing* down backwards... Yep, that is correct. Look at your graphic, starting from the Result, and go backwards to the Trigger. What happened right before you acted out? And, What happened right before that? ...And, What happened right before that? Noticing the answer to those questions, helps reveal what the cycle is, so it can be interrupted.

Roadblocks

We are going to break it down, going backward. At each phase of the cycle we are going to create *roadblocks* to prevent the behavior from happening again. This is good news! Call it a roadblock, barriers or blockades.

We will set up an off ramp around these to prevent the negative series of events from happening. Otherwise they progress (or get worse) in your life. Let us turn some things around.

Notice how the arrows in Figure 2.0 are heading back to the beginning. This is to signal your understanding, though it does not need to be drawn out. Notice how "roadblocks" 1-4 numbers go from right to left and from Result back to the original Trigger.

Figure 2.0 below is to get an idea of how we are going to structure the Freedom Protocol, starting with roadblock number 1 that conveniently looks like a stop sign! Okay, no mistake there!

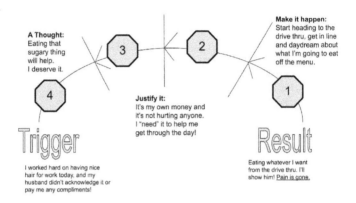

Figure 2.0
Freedom Protocol by Grace Revealed, LLC

Where Change Happens

Get excited! This is the good news in the process. At this point, we are going to start identifying the four roadblocks that can prevent the person in our example from acting out and emotionally eating whatever they want from the drive-thru. This next part of the process will help the person to navigate the painful feelings without the need to self-harm and dull the pain.

Some people may not need all 4 roadblocks, some may require more, but for this example it is helpful to understand how to break the self-sabotaging behaviors by having these 4 roadblocks set in place.

Picture This

A visual for you to picture is driving down the highway toward somewhere you do NOT belong and you know it is not good for you to go there! Then, you notice an off-ramp where you could take the exit and correct the course. The sign near the exit reads "Shit Show Highway ahead, next exit: Peace and Tranquility Boulevard"..

This process in the Freedom Protocol is the most successful way to break self-destructive, addictive, patterns and give you a plan for when you do get triggered. Please remember it's not if you get triggered, it is when the trigger happens. The trigger then becomes useful to alert you to use your self-care protocol. When your brain would normally self-sabotage, you take a different route.

Alright, enough about that! Let's get the plan started! Look at Figure 2.1 and follow along with your own plan. Remember we are here to help.

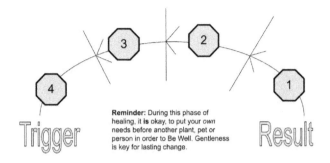

Figure 2.1
Freedom Protocol by Grace Revealed, LLC

Roadblock #1

Cancel the date! Cancel the order. Simply, apologize for getting in line at the drive-thru. Cancel it and get out of the line if you physically can. Do not pick it up at the pick-up window, get out of the line!

This can be useful for when you have something set up with a negative person, or you are trying to catch yourself from; using, gambling, drinking, watching pornography, or whatever the negative self-destructive drug of choice is.

<u>*NOTE: When the deed has not been done, you can still stop. There is hope.*</u>

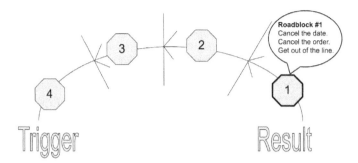

Figure 2.2
Freedom Protocol by Grace Revealed, LLC

Please reference figure 2.2 for an idea of what you are drawing on your own Freedom Protocol page. These steps are very important to work backward, from 1-4, right to left.

Roadblock #2

Make a call. At this stage in the process, picking up the phone can be a very productive and life-saving opportunity. It can feel VERY risky and vulnerable, but there **is** power in numbers. Telephone someone you trust. Call someone who will not judge you. Simply put, "tell on yourself". Tell on your brain. Let someone know that your brain is trying to destroy you! There is no shame in needing help.

Just sharing with someone that you *want help* is beneficial in itself. The listener may not be qualified to help you. The listener is helpful just by hearing about the pain you are in (the trigger). See Figure 2.3 for reference.

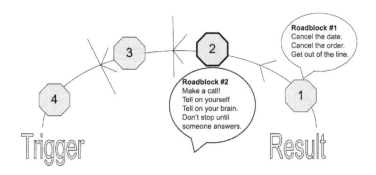

Figure 2.3
Freedom Protocol by Grace Revealed, LLC

Roadblock #3

Now is the time for some Truth Statements. Start to shower yourself with statements that are true. This is the time to remind ourselves that we want to be well! This is where self-talk can be a positive force for good. With our example, the lady could remind herself that she is valuable, wanted and beautiful, no matter what. She could remind herself that she's good enough and pleasing. She can remind herself that she is okay, no matter what. See Figure 2.4 for reference.

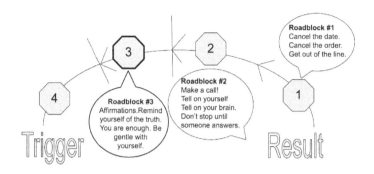

Figure 2.4
Freedom Protocol by Grace Revealed, LLC

Roadblock #4

Often roadblock number four could be instituted daily even before a trigger happens. We want to arm ourselves with beneficial processes that will help our brains heal from wounding. Then create new healthy patterns that will add value to our lives. Roadblock number four is preventative.

Now is the time to implement a self-care strategy that will help. This is where we check-in with four primary areas. HALT. Out of these four areas **H** is for Hungry. **A** is for Angry. **L** is for Lonely. And **T** is for Tired. A good question to ask ourselves at this point: Is one out of those 4 areas needing more attention than others? If so, primarily focus on tending to that one area first.

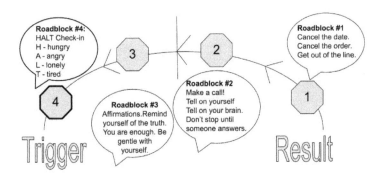

Figure 2.5
Freedom Protocol by Grace Revealed, LLC

Preventative Care

This is the time to take good care of yourself. When you are truly hungry, fix yourself a healthy life-giving meal, not a snack.

When you are angry, connect with someone who is equipped to talk through your circumstances and restore peace of mind. Before that anger rears its ugly head.

When you are lonely, and have been isolating (spending too much time by yourself), now is the time to socialize! Even when you feel like you have "no" friends. You can walk into a church. You can look up a Facebook group or a Meetup group that has something actively happening, in person, that day. You can find like-minded people to connect with. This is very important and does not happen overnight. Connecting with people in the flesh is crucial. Not an online group.

Lastly, when you are tired, please rest. When we are under-slept, it is a recipe for disaster. I give you permission to rest. Close your eyes. Set a timer for 5-10 minutes and take a nap. Set a timer for 20-60 minutes. Go to your car on a lunch break and rest your eyes. Give your body a chance to recuperate and reset.

Visual Reminders

For the visual learners out there: here are the visual representations of how to implement our 4 roadblocks again! Take a picture of it. If you don't need the visuals, feel free to glance and skip ahead.

FREEDOM PROTOCOL
Roadblocks to Recovery

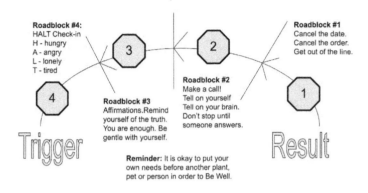

Figure 2.6
Freedom Protocol by Grace Revealed, LLC

REMINDER: It is okay to put your own needs before another plant, pet, or person in order to be well. Putting together a freedom protocol for yourself can be a challenge and we are here to help.

When you'd like some help executing your own personal **Freedom Protocol** visit GraceRevealedllc.com/book to schedule your 1-hour session and leave with a personalized Freedom Protocol plan to overcome past cycles! We are here to help you break free, once and for all.

Through engaging discussions and real-life examples, we explore the incredible benefits of embracing the Freedom Protocol. Imagine having a clear roadmap to follow when faced with triggers, enabling you to make empowered choices and break free from destructive habits. Experience the joy and confidence that comes from stepping into a life of freedom, unburdened by the chains of addiction.

Are you ready to embark on a journey of self-discovery and transformation? Visit www.gracerevealedllc.com/book to schedule your personal Freedom Protocol session today. Take the first step towards a life of liberation, where you can finally break free from the shackles of addictive patterns and embrace a future filled with limitless possibilities. Don't miss out on this life-changing experience! Unlock the key to your personal freedom with the Freedom Protocol by Grace Revealed LLC. Schedule your personal Freedom Protocol session and embark on a journey towards a life of liberation and empowerment. Remember, your freedom awaits!

Chapter 4 Summary:

In this chapter we talked about implementing strategies to break self-destructive patterns. We even walked through an example from being triggered to acting out and how to set up roadblocks to prevent those self-destructive patterns from happening. You now have a step-by-step guide to implement in your daily life. In addition, you now know where to turn for strategies for self-care when your own brain tempts you to self-sabotage.

In the chapters to come, we will talk about overcoming challenges and how to stay motivated in order to build resilience and overcome patterns. We will highlight tools for maintaining your transformation and ensuring your life improves. As you read on, we will look at reinstalling new, healthy, patterns that will bring you life! You will hear about systems to give you lasting peace of mind, no matter what. A sound mind.

CHAPTER 5

Handling Setbacks

Uncertainty

Okay! You are doing great. Hopefully by now, you have gained some awareness to *evaluate* your current circumstances, state of mind, and have a plan of how to implement the Freedom Protocol. But, now what? What about when the going gets tough? When you are having a bad day? When you are hungry, angry, lonely and tired?

This chapter is designed to acknowledge when challenges or setbacks arise. We will talk about what to do with the challenges, how to be proactive in order to stay motivated, and to bounce back quickly when problems arise.

We will discuss strategies for overcoming obstacles. You will hear inspiring stories of overcoming addiction. Ways to refuse to self-sabotage when all the odds seem to be against you. We will

...eking support and review how to build a supportive ...e will reinforce how important it is to be well.

...e is a question: What does it look like to have lasting peace of mind? It sounds something like this...

The Serenity Prayer
"God, grant me the serenity to accept the things I cannot change, courage to change the things I can, and wisdom to know the difference."

~Reinhold Nieburh

One of the greatest pieces in The Serenity Prayer is *acceptance* of the things we cannot change. Some big pieces in everyday life are that we cannot change: people, places, things and the weather of course! Sometimes life just happens. And, this book is here to give guidance to stay motivated and get back up when you feel like you're being crushed by circumstances. I get it, I have been through some of the unimaginable. Alas, here we are.

We are starting to understand how to get free, and sometimes pesky little demons try to come back to haunt us! Maybe for you, it is a flashback of a negative memory? Maybe, someone hurt you? Maybe, someone betrayed you or abandoned you when you needed them? Maybe it is a fear that is hard to shake? Maybe you just feel like giving up?

I assure you that Serenity is yours. By accepting the things we cannot change, we get ready to have courage to change the things that we can! The bonus part is having the wisdom to know the difference. Sometimes, we can simply call that; maturity.

Cannot Heal in the Same Environment that Makes Us Sick

Over the course of my healing journey, I have come to understand that we **cannot** heal in the same environment that made us sick. I hate to break it to you, although I am also grateful that I can expose that truth to you. When you are struggling and want to be well, you cannot heal in the same environment that made you sick. When you are ready to make some changes to be well, you may need to make difficult decisions to facilitate a healing environment.

Sometimes, we need to leave the environment we are in, that makes us sick, so that we can get to an environment that will make us well. For some of us, it might be a job change. For some of us, it might be a relationship change. For some of us, it might be a location change. For some it might mean leaving family members for a while. Change is not easy, but I assure you it is possible. Especially, when you want it and are willing to go to ANY length to be well.

Personal Story Time

I will never forget the time I was in the middle of a very big move. Going from one apartment to the next. Within the same

48-Hour timeframe, my dear friend and accountability partner went into a coma.

On top of that big move, and one of my best allies going into a coma, a man I thought I would marry dumped me! Ouch. Add some heartbreak to an already painfully stressful situation.

It is hard for me to put into words the unfathomable amount of emotional distress I was under during that time. Meanwhile, I was trying to "comprehend the word serenity", when I barely knew how to keep my life going. Trying to show up for my job, my family members, and wholeheartedly when it came to serving at church. I simply felt broken.

However, there was one thing I knew for sure! I knew, beyond a shadow of a doubt, I no longer wanted to numb the pain, escape, or self-sabotage during this incredibly difficult season of time. I remember telling myself over and over that "this too shall pass". "This too shall pass"... "this too shall pass"... Guess what? I made it through that very painful season.

And, it was the Freedom Protocol that got me through. Every morning I woke up and read *life giving* affirmations over myself. I washed my mind gently with scripture and statements of truth that I needed to hear. I planned my three meals a day, committed them to an accountability partner and ate them, no matter if I felt hungry or not. I wrote them down. I committed them to an accountability partner and I did not eat anything that would harm my body with food that season.

I committed to taking each day one hour at a time, and sometimes, one moment at a time. When I needed to cry, I cried. When I was feeling exhausted and fatigued, I rested. When I was feeling lonely, I made phone calls and I went to dinner parties. I painfully proclaimed "I had nothing to offer", except for the simple salad or healthy dish that I brought to share.

I gave myself permission to heal. I also gave myself permission to receive help from others. I received hugs, and sometimes I received awkward unhelpful advice from people that could not fathom the amount of emotional turmoil I was in.

One thing I remember is that having grace with myself was important. I am not perfect and I did not intend to be. I was a beautiful work in progress then, and I still am. One day at a time.

After studying many days, nights, weeks, months, and years about how the brain heals, I knew that I was putting myself in an environment that would make me well. I got around emotionally healthy people that did not try to "fix" or "rescue" me. I got around people that listened in order to understand me. They only offered loving suggestions when I welcomed them.

Studies have shown how magnificent our brains truly are scientifically! Numerous studies show how the brain can bounce back from painful experiences and heal. It has been proven that over time, new grooves can be made in it. Especially when we commit to *routines* that aid in our healing. When you simply commit to doing one day at a time of self-care, of healing, of stopping that self-sabotaging behavior, your brain *will* heal. Your brain will heal.

Another thing, please don't forget to celebrate your progress! Even when it feels like baby steps. Anything in the right direction is worth celebrating! In a healthy way. Maybe with a cup of coffee? Maybe with diet soda or maybe even with a new pillow or stuffed animal?

I am proud to say that I didn't give up during that extremely dark season when things felt hopeless for me; relationally, emotionally, and socially. As I stayed the course of well-being, things began to fall into place. After I reached the bottom of myself, and the most painful nights, I started to see the light at the end of the tunnel.

A Note of Hope: *Sometimes, the darkest nights give birth to the brightest breakthroughs! May that be encouragement to you as you venture through this life toward well-being! Healing is yours. Keep going.*

Soon after that season, I met my (now) husband. We got married within 6 months and moved into a home. I became a bonus mom to two young boys. Joy was restored!

I felt like I could catch my breath and I was walking the life that I was designed to live.. How? Because, I prioritize courage over comfort. I kept going in the face of adversity, because I wanted to be well. Beyond a shadow of a doubt.

Comfort is funny. After surviving over 30 years of compulsive overeating and comforting myself with food, I knew THAT was not an option for me. So, what would be an option? A person? No!

I needed to find *healthy* ways to soothe myself and find *comfort* that was not going to jeopardize my commitment to well-being. Here are some of the gifts of staying committed that give comfort and deeper healing to me:

- A cup of hot tea
- A 10-minute walk, without electronics
- Closing your eyes, in a comfortable position, for 5 to 10 minutes
- Having a good cry.
- Taking a hot bath and adding some epsom salts
- Planning ahead so you don't feel rushed
- Saying "No" when you feel depleted
- Being liberal with the thermostat. Enjoying the temperatures that your body craves
- Putting fruits, veggies and proteins first, to help think straight later

In the past, I would have felt inferior when I needed to ask for help. Help with finances? Help moving? Help with processing my thoughts? Help with a flat tire on the car? Help with a project at work? It is not always fun to ask for help.

We are living in a "self-taught" world since the expansion of the internet. With the gifts of Doctor Google, YouTube video tutorials, and other technology. There is still nothing more valuable on the planet than quality relationships and mentorship. Today, my ego can take a back seat. Asking someone for help is one of the most liberating things I've experienced in my adult life.

Supportive People Around Us

Now, let's shift gears and look at another important element of transformation. This helps with healing deeply, relationally. At this point in the book I want to talk about seeking support.

Building a supportive network around ourselves during the recovery process is a journey. Maybe, you're recovering from an isolated instance or injury. Maybe you're recovering from a lifetime of painful experiences? We may not ever know. Nevertheless, something I know to be true about healing from deep wounds is that the process of healing is expedited in the presence of those who *understand* and have walked the journey before us.

Sometimes it is nice to have a friend or family member who feels like they are supporting you, but I'd like to *challenge* this idea!

Let's talk about the value of finding a support group or a Social Circle. This would be a gathering of like-minded people who are committed to the same level of well-being, hobbies, self-development, or career focus that you are in.

When I have used the word "support network" in the past, it is easy for people to think about a *partner* or a *spouse* or a friend or a loved one. All too often, those people are *too close* to us and too close to our situations.. if that makes sense?

The closeness of a loved one makes it difficult for us to hear positive feedback and specific, quality directions. Especially when we are dealing with a sensitive matter. Hence, I encourage you to consider building or investing time into a supportive group that can add value to your healing journey. Ideally that you meet with on a Daily or Weekly basis. Where you leave feeling filled-up and encouraged.

These like-minded individuals can help with: overcoming challenges, building resilience, getting back up from hardship, asking for help, and setting healthy boundaries. A healthy support network helps with finding resources and will aid your ongoing journey. The journey to *live* your best life.

On the contrary, some "influencers" may leave you feeling depleted. Please avoid interactions with well-meaning people that drain your energy and leave you feeling wiped out. It is important to keep it simple.

Inside a valuable network of supportive people it can be really exciting to feel heard, known, and understood from those that "get" you. It is very important to be real with yourself and others. Also, it is important to know that you can't give what you don't have.

A simple search online of 12 step recovery groups (that value emotional sobriety) is a good place to start. A local networking group, church, or meet-up groups online that favor your area of need is ideal.

The best relationships are formed slowly over time, not rushed.

Chapter 5 Summary:

In this chapter we looked at overcoming challenges and building resilience. We talked about staying motivated and having some strategies for overcoming obstacles. We heard about enduring pain to get to the benefits of self-care, and we talked about having a supportive network around us.

In the upcoming chapter we will look at: how to re-organize our priorities, how to live with healthy boundaries, and to have nurturing healthy relationships. The kind of relationships that will support mental, emotional and spiritual health. Hang in there. You are doing great! Take a deep breath and I will see you in the next chapter.

CHAPTER 6

Balancing Boundaries

Living with Order

Welcome! glad you are here. You've come a long way! This chapter is about being well, staying well, how to live with *order* and avoid chaos. We will talk about how to re-organize our priorities and build healthy relationships with a framework of boundaries.

The boundaries will help us understand where we end and another person begins. We will look at support for mental, spiritual and emotional needs in order to be well. Some sage advice: trust the process. You *are* in the right place at the right time.

Introducing Boundaries

I'll never forget the time when I started exercising healthy boundaries. I'm not even sure I knew what boundaries *were* growing up in my family of origin. We had very loose boundaries in the home I emerged from as a youngster. Only when I went after my healing, did I discover that there is no such thing as "no boundaries". Besides the clothing brand at Walmart. No Boundaries is not a real thing.

Types of Boundaries

There are three different types of boundaries that families typically exhibit. Loose boundaries, strict or rigid boundaries, and healthy balanced boundaries. We will get into that in this chapter!

Loose Boundaries: Loose boundaries refer to a style of boundary-setting where individuals have difficulty asserting their own needs and limits. People with loose boundaries often find it challenging to say "no" and may feel overwhelmed by the demands and expectations of others. They may prioritize the needs of others over their own, leading to feelings of resentment or being taken advantage of. This lack of clear boundaries can result in a loss of personal identity and a sense of being controlled by external influences.

Rigid Boundaries: Rigid boundaries, on the other hand, involve an excessive level of strictness and inflexibility. Individuals with rigid boundaries tend to have a strong need for control and may have difficulty forming close relationships. They often have a fear of being vulnerable and may keep others at a distance emotionally. Rigid boundaries can lead to isolation and a lack of intimacy, as well as difficulties in adapting to new situations or accepting different perspectives. It's important to note that rigid boundaries can be a defense mechanism to protect oneself from potential harm or emotional pain.

Healthy Boundaries: Healthy boundaries are a balanced approach to setting limits and maintaining personal autonomy while respecting the needs and boundaries of others. Individuals with healthy boundaries have a clear understanding of their own values, beliefs, and limits. They can assert their needs and desires without feeling guilty or selfish, while also respecting the boundaries of others. Healthy boundaries promote healthy relationships, as they allow for open communication, mutual respect, and the ability to prioritize self-care. They provide a sense of security, allowing individuals to maintain their own identity while engaging in meaningful connections with others.

Remember, boundaries are not fixed and can vary depending on the situation and the individuals involved. It's important to regularly assess and adjust your boundaries to ensure they align with your values and promote your overall well-being.

Practicing Boundaries

As I was attempting to understand how to implement healthy boundaries, I started to have little whispers come to my mind. The "whispers" sounded like this.. "Start with making your bed and your mind will follow". Did you hear that? "Make your bed and your mind will follow". Then, I heard statements like, "Take care of your mind and your body will follow.

Oh man! My brain started having strong reactions toward attempting to make my bed in the morning. I was used to a high level of chaos in my life. Exercising healthy boundaries with myself for the first time seemed daunting.

So I timed it! It took somewhere between 30 seconds and 2 minutes to make my bed, depending on how many sheets, blankets and pillows that were there, any given season. That's not too long! 30 seconds to 2 minutes! If you're not already doing it, I encourage you to start making your bed, as soon as you wake up in the morning. Even before using the bathroom. It is truly a game changer. When I got comfortable with setting boundaries, I could feel myself being set free.

If we want order in our minds, we have to have order in our surroundings. Funny how it works both ways. When we have order in our surroundings, we start to have order in our minds! Test it out for yourself!

The Landscape of the Mind

Have you ever felt like you just can't get a handle on your own brain? Sometimes our brains do funny things! And, I assure you that taking little baby steps, to put order to things around you, will have a lasting effect on the landscape of your mind.

Picture this:

Close your eyes for a moment and picture what the landscape inside your brain looks like, today. Is it a well maintained garden? Has your garden been weeded and pruned? Or are there boxes and bags all over the place? Does the trash need to be taken out? Are you letting people see the real you?

Take a moment to capture the picture of what things look like in the landscape of your mind today. Consider jotting it down or drawing a picture. There is a powerful force of love that wants you to experience the fullness of life. When we are ready to receive the fullness of life, we often need to let go of things that are not serving our well-being. This has been proven time and time again in the history of mankind.

The Law of Sowing and Reaping

In the context of inner healing, the Law of Sowing and Reaping suggests that the thoughts, emotions, and behaviors we cultivate within ourselves will have an impact on our overall well-being and personal growth. If we sow positive thoughts, self-compassion, and healthy behaviors, we are more likely to reap positive outcomes and experience inner healing.

Conversely, if we sow negative thoughts, self-destructive behaviors, or hold onto unresolved emotional wounds, we may experience negative consequences and hinder our inner healing process. These negative patterns can manifest as recurring negative emotions, self-sabotaging behaviors, or difficulties in forming healthy relationships.

To apply the Law of Sowing and Reaping to inner healing, it is important to cultivate self-awareness and take responsibility for our thoughts, emotions, and actions. By consciously choosing to sow positive seeds, such as self-love, forgiveness, gratitude, and personal growth, we can create a fertile ground for inner healing to take place.

It's important to note that inner healing is a journey that requires time, patience, and self-compassion. The Law of Sowing and Reaping reminds us that the efforts we put into our inner healing process will yield results over time. By consistently sowing positive seeds and making choices that align with our healing and growth, we can gradually transform our inner landscape and experience greater emotional well-being.

Remember, inner healing is a deeply personal process, and it can be beneficial to seek support from therapists, coaches, or mentors who can provide guidance and tools to navigate this journey.

Here is an idea: Start with your mind and your body will follow. Start making your bed and your mind will follow. Implement small measures of putting more order to your surroundings and your brain will thank you.

Once you put order to the wonderful mind you've been given, more order will follow. It is true, we reap what we sow. It is a law that all humans live by, whether we like it or not.

How about this? When we sow into *order* we will reap *order*. On the flip side, when we sew into chaos, we reap chaos. When we sow into abundance, we reap abundance. When we sow into scarcity we reap scarcity. This law of the universe is a simple truth. Maybe you needed a gentle reminder of that fact today?

Revelations come in order to correct-course on how our life looks today, so we can have a better tomorrow! Mull over this awareness when you consider what you want life to look like tomorrow, the next day, month, year, 5 years, or even 10 years from now.

The Importance of Supportive Connections

I will never forget the year that a very special couple came into my life. They had "adopted" me spiritually, and with their time, energy and love. One weekend at home I was crying and trying to let go of my painful past when I got a knock on the door. I was greeted with a bouquet of white roses and two visitors. I don't know exactly how it happened except that they were on a "special assignment" to love me back to life from the rubble I had left in my rearview mirror.

During that time, I had felt like giving up. I had felt like I had completely ruined my life. I was a walking train wreck of bad decisions. My romantic "picker" was broken and I didn't know how to make healthy decisions. I had worked myself to the point of burnout and my body and organs were starting to shut down.

Somehow, this very special couple decided that they wanted to love me *without* an agenda. They willingly spent time to hear what was on my heart. They offered feedback, only when I was open to it or asking for their advice. They heard me. They loved me and they offered support when I was willing to receive it.

During that season, the acceptance that I felt was beyond anything I had ever experienced. You could not put a monetary value on it. Any book I read, any training I had gone to, any prayer I had ever prayed, could not compare to the feeling of love and acceptance that I felt when I was with them.

Let's call them The Blessing. The Blessing put me on a wavelength to receive support in a way I had never experienced in my adult life before. The notable thing here is that I didn't go looking for it. Although, I did welcome the support I needed, and let God do the rest!

It is so important to be surrounded by loving people that don't try to "fix" or "rescue" you. I've met a lot of "fixers" and "rescuers" in my day. Unfortunately they don't do much good. They do not seem to understand that they are *enabling* people by attempting to do things for them. The best support comes from those who encourage people to overcome their challenges with their own strength. They are like a spotter that says "you got this", "one more rep" and "you can do it!".

Building healthy relationships during a recovery journey takes time and effort. It takes open communication. It takes building trust and mutual respect. Building healthy relationships is a journey in and of itself. And, there is a starting point.

When you want a beginning, a starting point, I encourage you that it starts with us! Ourselves. You. We cannot have healthy relationships with others if we do not have a healthy relationship with ourselves. What I also discovered is - in order for me to have a healthy relationship with myself I needed to have a healthy relationship with God.

In no way is this a religious book. I don't have time or interest in writing about *that*. Although, it is important to share that healing in the mind, body and spirit is somewhat of a *supernatural* experience. It takes more than will-power and human strength.

Sometimes God uses nature. Like flowers, smells, mountain hikes, trails and greenery. Sometimes it could be the smile of a young child to set us free from inner turmoil! Healing is supernatural.

Exercising Healthy Boundaries

Within healthy relationships, there exists healthy boundaries. Knowing where I end and another person begins. Physical boundaries are the first to come to mind with the visual of a physical beginning and ending to our bodies. These boundaries involve touch. For example; whether or not to give or receive a hug. Hugs should never be taken, forced, or stolen.

If you've ever had that happen to you (someone stealing a hug), then you know that it is uncomfortable! Never be afraid to set a touch boundary. Touch should always be consensual. Where touch is offered and welcomed.

Occasionally, you have to set *listening* boundaries also. Over the years, I discovered that people enjoy "opening up" when they feel safe to share "anything". However, it may not always be "safe" for the listener to hear the other person's pain.

It is okay to simply say something like this. "Thank you for trusting me with delicate information, but I'd prefer to stay focused on the positive outcome over the painful details. Maybe another listener is more suitable than me. Thanks for understanding where I am coming from". And leave it there.

How about financial boundaries? How about emotional boundaries? Or when or when not to visit boundaries? How long to stay when visiting? There are lots of great teachings on boundaries and this is just a brief glance at exercising healthy boundaries.

One observation I've seen among hurting people trying to heal is this grave misunderstanding. They think setting boundaries is for the other person. In reality, setting boundaries is truly only for the individual who sets them.

I must set boundaries for **my** well-being, not for yours. And that is completely okay. Saying "no" to something or someone to protect your peace of mind is a decision that is well worth making. The power of "no". Giving away your peace of mind and sanity to "please" another person will only end up feeling bankrupt, lost, and confused. Empty.

Boundaries are important for maintaining protection. Mental, physical, and emotional protection from toxic people is of utmost importance. There can be people in our "sphere" who tempt us to give away our emotional energy or *peace of mind* because they have different boundaries than us, loose boundaries.

Maintaining healthy boundaries creates a supportive environment for us to *heal* from self-destructive patterns, and gain emotional sobriety. One day at a time and one instance at a time. Ongoing peace of mind is available to each of us when we are willing to work toward the simplicity of maintaining our own boundaries. However, there are things that can hold us back from living a simple care-free life. They are burdens.

Letting Go

Burdens come in different forms and from different sources. As a woman, I know there are many facets to life that tempt me to get overwhelmed, worried and anxious. Instead of focusing on the negative burdens that hold us back, we can look at a solution to be free of them!

An extremely powerful way to feel *lighter*; mentally, physically and emotionally **is** to *let go* of my burdens! Maybe you're wondering how to do that? Maybe you are questioning, am I able to let go?

Letting go of emotional pain is a process that involves acknowledging, accepting, and releasing the negative emotions that are holding us back. Here are some steps that can help in the process:

Acknowledge the pain: The first step is to recognize and acknowledge the emotional pain you are experiencing. This involves being honest with yourself about your feelings and allowing yourself to fully experience them without judgment. It's important to give yourself permission to feel and validate your emotions.

Understand the pain: Take time to explore the root causes and triggers of your emotional pain. Reflect on the events, experiences, or relationships that have contributed to your pain.

This self-reflection can help you gain insight into the patterns and beliefs that may be perpetuating the pain.

Acceptance and forgiveness: Acceptance is a crucial step in the process of letting go. It involves acknowledging that the past cannot be changed and that holding onto pain only prolongs suffering. Practice self-compassion and forgiveness, both towards yourself and others involved. Remember that forgiveness does not mean condoning or forgetting, but rather releasing the emotional burden that comes with holding onto resentment or anger.

Release and express emotions: Find healthy ways to release and express your emotions. This can include journaling, talking to a trusted friend or therapist, engaging in creative outlets like art or music, or practicing mindfulness and meditation. Allow yourself to express your emotions in a safe and supportive environment.

Cultivate self-care and self-love: Prioritize self-care activities that nourish your mind, body, and soul. Engage in activities that bring you joy, relaxation, and peace. Practice self-compassion and self-love by treating yourself with kindness, patience, and understanding.

Reframe and reframe your narrative: Challenge negative thought patterns and beliefs that may be perpetuating your emotional pain. Replace them with positive and empowering thoughts. Focus on personal growth, resilience, and the lessons learned from your experiences.

Seek support: It can be helpful to seek support from a therapist, counselor, or support group. They can provide guidance, tools, and a safe space to explore and heal emotional pain. Surround yourself with a supportive network of friends and loved ones who can offer understanding and encouragement.

Remember, letting go of emotional pain is a process that takes time and patience. Be gentle with yourself and allow yourself to heal at your own pace. Each person's journey is unique, and what works for one may not work for another. Trust in your ability to heal and embrace the transformative power of letting go.

Wherever you are *in the process* of letting go of mental and emotional baggage, I assure you that letting go **is** possible. Part of my role as a professional is to test theories and prove their credibility or deny them. Over the past several years, I had a *hunch* that **when** people let go of emotional, mental and spiritual burdens that their *physical* bodies would get lighter. Guess what? They do!

Men and women's bodies do indeed change when they face what was holding them back. When people go through a process of letting go (of mental, spiritual, and emotional baggage), their shoulders sit back, they stand tall again, and their bodies start to lose weight. Time after time.

Emotional Freedom

Emotional pain is burdensome. Spiritual wounding is heavy. Mental torment is weighty. Some of us sabotage ourselves and some of us let someone else torment us. Pain is funny like that.

If you're still reading this book and you've made it this far, I assure you that there is freedom available that will help you feel lighter and truly live better. When you "trust the process" and stop trying to "go it alone" or "figure it out" all by yourself. Positive growth and transformation can happen freely.

Another truism I've found in decades of research; healing actually takes place deeply and more quickly **with** support of others rather than trying to "go it alone". At Grace Revealed, it is an honor to watch people's lives transform in front of us. Sometimes, it is one soul at a time. Sometimes it is a small group at a time, and sometimes it is a corporation undergoing transformation. You will find a safe haven with Grace Revealed workshops, wellness programs, and coaching that allow you to *let go* of pain and be restored. You can be made new on this journey called life. Restoration is yours!

Enemies of Change

There is a proven path toward healing that I discovered and you can too. The path is simpler than a person may think, but there is also an enemy to that path. That enemy sometimes comes in the form of whispering lies, a charming partner, our own thoughts. When it comes to change and transformation, there are several common enemies that can hinder progress. Here are a few examples:

Fear: Fear is a powerful emotion that can hold us back from embracing change. Fear of the unknown, fear of failure, or fear of stepping outside our comfort zones can prevent us from taking the necessary steps towards transformation. Recognizing and addressing our fears is essential in overcoming them and moving forward.

Resistance to discomfort: Change often involves stepping into unfamiliar territory and facing discomfort. Our natural inclination is to seek comfort and avoid discomfort. However, growth and transformation require us to embrace discomfort and push through it. Resisting discomfort can keep us stuck in old patterns and prevent us from experiencing personal growth.

Lack of self-belief: Believing in ourselves and our ability to change is crucial for transformation. If we doubt our capabilities or have a negative self-image, it becomes challenging to make meaningful changes. Cultivating self-belief and practicing self-compassion can help overcome this enemy and foster a mindset of growth.

Attachment to the past: Holding onto the past, whether it's past mistakes, regrets, or outdated beliefs, can hinder our ability to move forward. Letting go of what no longer serves us and embracing the present moment is essential for transformation. It requires a willingness to release attachments and open ourselves up to new possibilities.

Lack of support: Trying to navigate change and transformation alone can be challenging. Surrounding ourselves with a supportive network of friends, family, or mentors who believe in our potential can make a significant difference. They can provide encouragement, guidance, and accountability, helping us stay motivated and committed to our transformational journey.

Fixed mindset: Having a fixed mindset, where we believe our abilities and qualities are fixed traits, can limit our potential for change. Embracing a growth mindset, on the other hand, allows us to see challenges as opportunities for growth and believe in our capacity to learn and evolve. Adopting a growth mindset opens up possibilities for transformation.

Lack of clarity and direction: Without a clear vision or goals, it can be challenging to initiate and sustain change. Setting clear intentions and defining what we want to achieve through transformation provides a sense of direction and purpose. It helps us stay focused and motivated during the process.

It's important to remember that these enemies of change are common and normal. Recognizing them is the first step in overcoming them. By cultivating self-awareness, seeking support, and embracing a growth mindset, we can navigate these challenges and embark on a transformative journey.

Yes, that *saboteur* can be our own thoughts, or a flat out evil person with their own best interest at heart. Letting go of pain can often be messy -but I assure you- it is worth going down the uncomfortable path that leads to joy, peace and prosperity. One day at a time.

Please consider this for awareness, and something to stay mindful of, on your journey of healing. This is not to scare you, but bring awareness to the fact that we need to safeguard our healing. We especially need to safeguard our healing during the first 90 days of letting go of old behaviors and compulsive patterns. Gentleness and awareness are simply tools to help the healing process.

Try this:

In your notebook or journal, jot down a few burdens OR enemies of change that you would like to let go of. Picture the enemy or burdens you wrote down. Visualize, physically throwing them into a rushing waterfall and letting them go, never to pick them up again!

Then, once you can physically feel the burden leaving your body, mentally push these burdens over the waterfall. Then stop, wait for a moment and receive whatever blessing that comes in place of what once was that burden. It is a worthy trade.

Is it joy? Feel the joy! Is it peace of mind? Let the Peace wash over your mind! Do this as often as you like, until you feel like you have let go of everything you needed to and replaced it with something better.

Chapter 6 Summary:

Let's summarize this chapter and get ready to move forward with well-being! In this chapter we talked about living with order. We are taking steps to prepare ourselves for healthy relationships inside the context of healthy boundaries. We looked at types of boundaries and what healthy boundaries look like. We talked about the role of boundaries and we talked about letting go of past hurt. We talked about the enemy of change and staying alert.

Stay connected with us at GraceRevealedLLC.com and I look forward to seeing you at an upcoming event, an online or in-person workshop!

CHAPTER 7

Emotional Sobriety

You Are The Miracle

If you've made it this far, then you are a living miracle! At this point you may be wondering.. is it really *that* simple? I'm used to turbulence, anxiety, and feeling overwhelmed. Can I really live with emotional sobriety and peace of mind on a regular basis? Yes, it really is that simple. This should come as a relief.

When we have a personal Freedom Protocol set in place, then it doesn't matter what the trigger is, we can override our brains and implement our own protocol, one instance at a time. One topic at a time. We are strengthened with the support of others who can lovingly take a call and help keep us accountable to our commitment of well-being. Over the years of prioritizing recovery, a certain pattern of human behavior has shown through that I don't hear many people talk about. Drama.

Drama refers to a pattern of seeking out or creating chaotic or emotionally charged situations in our lives. It can become a habitual way of seeking excitement, validation, or a sense of control. However, this addiction to drama can be detrimental to our emotional well-being and relationships. It is the subtle addiction that no one talks about.

Addicted to Excitement

There was a time when I knew I was addicted to excitement and every day was another opportunity for *drama* in my life. There was a limited amount of space for peace and a sound mind. Because I was so addicted to chaos and people pleasing it seemed hard to relinquish those negative behaviors in exchange for positive stable behaviors.

I knew it was an "inside job". If I wanted to change the *fruit* in my life, I had to look at the *root* in my life. Facing my childhood trauma and the dynamics of my dysfunctional family of origin shed much light on *where to begin* with the healing process.

I no longer wanted to live with constant drama and emotional stimulation and toxicity. I wanted peace. I prayed for the 3 W's (the willingness to be willing to be willing). I prayed to accept the things I cannot change, for courage to change the things that I could, and wisdom to know the difference. I prayed to keep an open mind, to try things beyond what I normally would. Get out of my comfort zone.

This changed everything! This cracked the code in my own life to live with emotional sobriety. Week after week, a "safe setting" was shown to me. Where I could process where I came from. Sometimes it was with a support group, sometimes my therapist, other times a clinical intensive workshop. I was willing to go to *any* length to be well and change.

This helped me discover the path out of complex PTSD. At other times, it was with hugs from little children and knowing eye contact from members in the rooms of 12-step recovery. The recovery rooms of Adult Children of Alcoholics & Dysfunctional Families.

Other times, it happened in the rooms of Sex and Love Addiction to overcome my intimacy disorder. We never can tell exactly what will come to help heal us. But, I promise you, it will come, when you are open, honest and willing. True humility is an advantage over cosmetic humility.

Admitting a need for help takes truth strength and courage. Take the courage you have, let go and see what happens next.

The work of transformation is not for the weak of heart. At times, you may get discouraged and have to encourage yourself to keep going. It will be worth it. You now have an arsenal of tools to succeed. Will you be the next story of amazing transformation and change? Cry a little if you need to. Have a big ugly cry when you need to. Being uncomfortable for a season. See hardship as the pathway to peace. It gives birth to a new you.

Emotional Sobriety

Emotional sobriety is making a commitment to love ourselves and be good to ourselves. We stop harming ourselves by attaining emotional sobriety and replacing harm with care. By using this definition we set the stage for significance in the recovery process.

We have emotional awareness today and we are committed to regulating our emotions and learning from them. No longer do we have to disconnect from ourselves and others when pain arises. We can feel and heal.

Emotional sobriety is achieved by starting with a decision in our minds before any action takes place. We can decide to be a *good parent* to our inner child who was abandoned, neglected or rejected. Those feelings... Those painful feelings we experienced in childhood carry into adult experiences if they were not properly loved and healed. Will you make a commitment to love and be good to yourself from this day forward?

Step one of the 12 Steps states that we are powerless. Being able to admit that I was powerless over my painful reactions to everyday situations was important. If you read this far you have taken on a challenging journey to live a life full of serenity, a sound mind, and even childlike joy!

It is time to embrace yourself. Embrace all the ups and downs that you have been through, embrace the pain of letting go and celebrate yourself for coming this far. You have boundaries today! You have a plan to handle triggers and bumps in the road that tempt you to give away your serenity, you are a smashing success as you put your well-being first, one day at a time.

I want to give you permission to lighten up. I give you permission to play. I give you permission to enjoy life!

Long-term Sanity

One of the chief ways to maintain peace of mind is to have *no* agenda, to make *no* assumptions, and to live life as it comes. Practicing gratitude gives light to the lessons we learn from pain. Acceptance, letting go and the practice of forgiveness brings lasting stability and peace of mind. It is okay to settle into serenity. No one is going to steal it from you today. Peace of mind is yours.

As your journey unfolds, you will likely have an opportunity to forgive others for the pain they contributed that hurt you. One promise in the healing journey I've discovered is that "hurt people, hurt people" and healed people, heal people. As you become well and heal at the deepest level possible, you will help heal others!

Emotional sobriety attracts other emotionally stable people and it repels people that are toxic. As you up your commitment to being emotionally stable, your tolerance for unstable people may need some loving adjustments. You will be able to effectively communicate healthy boundaries and intuitively know how to communicate what you need within healthy relationships. You will be able to resolve conflict more effectively. You will become a better *listener* and more empathetic to others who are in pain. You will be able to foster healthy connections as you let petty differences fade away and be able to focus on solutions rather than dwelling on problems.

Emotional healing is not necessarily something that can be bought, but it can be seen by the ripple effects in all areas of your life. Examples are: financial stability, emotional stability, mental stability, and physical health. These are all byproducts of putting healing first. You will make more meaningful connections with others and be able to navigate crises more effectively.

When you stay in a lifestyle of the Serenity Prayer; "God, grant me the serenity to accept the things I cannot change, courage to change the things I can, and the wisdom to know the difference", lasting peace and stability become a reality and not just a fancy idea.

Try this:

Next time you are in a situation that tempts you to panic, look at your Freedom Protocol and *remember that no one can steal your serenity*. Try journaling and answering the journal questions on your bookmark for at least 14 days straight! Can you do it? Stay close to the Grace Revealed LLC community and see what other levels of healing you will get to, when you put yourself first.

Chapter 7 Summary:

In this chapter we looked at the benefits of emotional sobriety, defined what it is and what it looks like in our lives. We talked about long-term serenity over excitement and drama. You are encouraged to remain childlike and let healing unfold. Venture into the last chapter to hear about getting well, staying well and living an extraordinary life you were meant to live!

CHAPTER 8

Get Well, Be Well, Stay Well

Wellness

Okay! You have put in the hard work and now it is time to maintain your long-term recovery by walking well. You are restored. You get to be restored, renewed, and transformed into the magnificent man or woman that you were designed to be!

By now, you have figured out that many things have tempted you to give up, but you kept going. In the next few pages we are going to explore alternative ways to manage emotions, stress, and challenges. Without resorting to addictive self-sabotaging behaviors. What will life look like when we are walking free?

In this chapter we are going to talk about The Beautiful Exchange. We are going to talk about building a new foundation for well-being. We are going to talk about the reward of you being yourself! We are going to talk about strategies for maintaining emotional sobriety. We are going to talk about healthy coping mechanisms and we are going to talk about a plan for moving forward. Are you ready?

Let's not forget about those very important ingredients we mentioned earlier: desire to change, willingness, and courage to try something we've never tried before! Let's dig in.

Question: Do You Want to Be Well?

If I gave you a brick of gold today, what would you do to protect it?

When we work to become well, we want you to keep the valuable treasures we have worked to obtain. In this chapter, you will hear suggestions for healthy outlets such as hobbies, creative expression, and support groups to aid in long-term recovery.

A gentle reminder: this is not a once-and-done journey. This is ongoing, and it *is* a process. Just because it takes time doesn't mean it's not good. Remember the idea of delayed gratification?

Delayed Gratification

Delayed gratification refers to the ability to resist immediate rewards or pleasures in order to achieve a greater, long-term benefit or goal. It involves exercising self-control and patience by choosing to forgo immediate gratification in favor of a more desirable outcome in the future.

Here are a few examples to illustrate delayed gratification:

Saving money: Instead of spending money on impulse purchases or immediate desires, you choose to save and invest your money for future financial security or to achieve a specific goal, such as buying a house or starting a business.

Healthy lifestyle choices: Opting for nutritious meals and regular exercise instead of indulging in unhealthy foods or sedentary behaviors. By prioritizing long-term health and well-being, you delay the immediate pleasure of unhealthy habits for the greater reward of improved physical fitness and overall health.

Academic or professional pursuits: Spending time studying, researching, or honing your skills instead of engaging in leisure activities. By dedicating time and effort to your education or career, you delay immediate leisure or entertainment to achieve long-term success and personal growth.

Building relationships: Investing time and energy in building meaningful relationships rather than seeking instant gratification through casual encounters. By nurturing and developing deeper connections with others, you delay immediate gratification for the long-term rewards of companionship, support, and emotional fulfillment.

Entrepreneurial endeavors: Starting a business or pursuing a passion project requires delayed gratification. It often involves investing time, resources, and effort upfront without immediate financial rewards. By persevering through the initial challenges and delays, you work towards the long-term goal of building a successful venture or realizing your creative vision.

Delayed gratification can be challenging, as it requires discipline and the ability to resist immediate temptations. However, it can lead to greater personal growth, achievement, and fulfillment in the long run. By practicing delayed gratification, you develop resilience, patience, and the ability to prioritize long-term goals over short-term pleasures.

Moving Forward

Healthy relationships add value that are beyond monetary value. We will talk about building the right support around you during your transformation that is the best for you. Only you can gauge that, although we will offer some suggestions in this chapter.

Remember the visual in the beginning of the book with the construction site? We want to talk about the mending process in this chapter. The land has been cleared, the old junk has been exposed, some walls have been knocked down, and we are ready to start restoring sanity. A whole, brand new person is ready to emerge. The house has been restored. It may be on the same land, but it is not the same house. It has been completely renovated and it has tripled in value!

Do you see it in your mind's eye? This is important for your personal journey to understand where you are in the process. Maybe you already did a lot of work before you picked up this book? Maybe you've lived through a couple of those negative cycles and haven't been able to break the self-sabotage cycle. Maybe you've worked really hard white knuckling to stop yourself from negative addictive patterns.

Healing is organic, I can't begin to guess at the pain that you have had to overcome before you were led to this book. When you put into practice some of the suggestions in this book, you will know happiness and you will know peace. But my challenge to you today is what are you willing to do to protect it? To maintain it? Or maybe to enhance it even further?

Are you willing to keep going when the going gets rough? When the world seems to conspire against you? If you have the grit, determination, and willingness to keep trying (even when everything inside you is crying to give up) you are in the right place!

Maybe for a time you had to break away from; other people, your job, your living situation, maybe even your children, or loved ones? As we recover from difficult situations there comes a time where we may need to re-engage others again. Maybe you need to make amends? Or maybe you need to go back to work, but as a new person? As someone who is working to take responsibility for themselves and to heal deeply.

In this chapter we will talk about how to re-engage our lives as we know it. I want to start with a couple simple affirmations:

Number one, **you are enough**. Secondly, you are right *on time* for *your* healing. You are right on time for a better life.

If you've had the opportunity to see a reconstruction project or a home renovation or any type of construction site.. things get messy! But, my goodness, what a feeling it is to see the finished product!

While the stages of a major renovation building project are specific to construction, we can draw parallels between these stages and the process of personal transformation. Here's how they can be related:

Planning and Design: In personal transformation, this stage involves setting clear goals and objectives for the changes you want to make in your life. It includes self-reflection, identifying areas for growth, and creating a plan or vision for your transformation.

Pre-construction: This stage is akin to preparing yourself for personal transformation. It involves gathering resources, seeking support from mentors or coaches, and creating a supportive environment that aligns with your goals. It may also involve addressing any limiting beliefs or emotional barriers that could hinder your progress.

Demolition and Site Preparation: In personal transformation, this stage represents letting go of old patterns, beliefs, and behaviors that no longer serve you. It involves releasing negative emotions, shedding self-limiting beliefs, and creating space for new possibilities and growth.

Construction: This stage is where the actual work of personal transformation takes place. It involves implementing new habits, acquiring new skills, and making changes in your thoughts, behaviors, and actions. It requires consistent effort, discipline, and perseverance to build the foundation for personal growth.

MEP Installations: Just as mechanical, electrical, and plumbing installations are essential for a functional building, personal transformation requires addressing the core aspects of your life. This includes improving your mental and emotional well-being, enhancing your relationships, and nurturing your physical health.

Finishes and Interior Work: This stage represents the refinement and fine-tuning of your personal transformation. It involves developing self-awareness, practicing self-care, and cultivating positive habits and mindsets. It also includes integrating new learnings and insights into your daily life.

Final Touches and Completion: In personal transformation, this stage signifies the culmination of your efforts. It involves celebrating your progress, acknowledging your achievements, and embracing the transformed version of yourself. It also includes ongoing maintenance and continuous growth to sustain the positive changes you've made.

By relating the stages of a major renovation building project to personal transformation, we can understand that personal growth requires careful planning, preparation, and consistent effort. It involves letting go of old patterns, implementing new habits, and refining ourselves to create a more fulfilling and meaningful life.

Remember, personal transformation is a unique and individual journey. It's important to be patient, kind to yourself, and seek support when needed. Embrace the process and enjoy the progress you make along the way.

Where things were once on paper, now they are in real life! They are enhanced, transformed and renovated with a new look. Let that be a gauge for where you are in the process of healing and transformation. Take a moment to check in with yourself to gauge where you're at in the process above. What stage of reconstruction are you in?

As I was practicing the process of letting go of the old behaviors and patterns which were no longer serving me, I realized something. I needed to know WHAT I would receive in return. If I was going to let go of these things that once got me through seasons of hardship, I needed to see the reward. What would

I actually gain by releasing these negative patterns? And, the Beautiful Exchange emerged.

The Beautiful Exchange

The Beautiful Exchange is when we **let go** of something *harmful* for something *helpful*. This is the process where we let go of junk for something better. We exchange fear for hope, we exchange hopelessness for faith. We exchange bitterness to be better. We leave feeling helpless and become helpful. We leave negative self-talk and gain self-affirmations and truthfulness. We give up pleasing people and gain a sense of belonging. We ask for help when we would normally try to be self-reliant. We let go of burdens and gain blessings. We invite the new as we let go of the old!

New Foundations

When we build a new foundation, we cannot try to put the old crap back into the new concrete. We have to actually let it be a new foundation. So what does a new foundation look like emotionally, mentally, or spiritually? Well.. how is the new house built? Brick by brick, piece by piece. The more intentional each piece, the stronger the house will be.

I remember helping a dear friend build their home in the Adirondack Mountains. It was bitter cold when we decided to frame the home and build a two-story house in the middle of winter. In this age of instant gratification, it felt like it took us forever to accomplish anything!

The interesting thing I learned about the building process was that each phase takes time because of the deliberate action that each phase requires. There is a time when things are framed in order to prepare for the right size of windows and doors. There is a time when the walls are left open to prepare for electrical and plumbing. There is a time when there is a hole between each of the levels while the stair stringers are being constructed. There is a time without a roof while the tresses are being engineered and installed. There is a time of bare walls before final paint colors are selected. There is a time of darkness before the lights are installed and the electricity is turned on. There is a time of bone chilling temperatures before the warmth of a loving family can be felt. There was a time and a season for all of it. Please keep the process in mind as you are allowing yourself to heal from negative, self-destructive patterns.

Another phrase I heard in the 12-step rooms of recovery was "you're only as sick as your secret". What does that mean, exactly? Does that mean I'm hiding something? Lying to myself? Lying to someone else? What kind of secrets did I have that were making me sick? Some quality questions to ask yourself on a journey of deeper healing. Especially, when you are choosing to Be well and stay well.

Emotional sobriety relies on a level of integrity and honesty that cannot be jeopardized by the slightest untruth.

In my journey of recovery I have been tempted to withhold information from others that are deserving of the truth. That made me sick. Physically sick, emotionally sick and mentally ill. I was in need of a trustworthy person to disclose my hidden truth to, safely.

Something to consider here is finding a person who will not judge or offer feedback without request. Just a listening ear will do. Who we entrust the *whole* truth to *does* matter greatly! Please take caution with who you share, when a deep secret needs to come out of you.

Wondering how to decide? Here are a couple questions to ask ourselves. Have they proven their trustworthiness? Are our secrets safe with them? Some of us have been through some very painful and traumatic experiences. There are listening ears out there who are willing to use our truth against us. A word of discernment to only share with those who have proven that they are *safe* with delicate information. Choose wisely.

Maintenance.

Let's talk about maintenance! As many layers of the past fall off of us, a new life is born. Sometimes it is fragile, like a baby, and needs a lot of care to protect from going back to where we came from. I encourage you to stay solution minded when you are up against a temptation to go backwards.

I'll never forget the visual of an old farmhouse I saw on the side of the road on a long road trip. I can only imagine it was a beautiful house back in its day. Over time, it got ignored and no one continued to maintain it. On the other hand, we could drive by old mansions that were well maintained because someone cared for them and took care of the doors, windows, roof, siding, and all the landscaping around the property.

Maintenance gives the home its glory! Maintenance takes consistency and a value on preserving the goodness of the home. I implore you to take this into consideration as transformation happens inside of you.

When the inside changes and becomes more free of pain, the outside will reflect the inner change. Please continue to take good care of yourself and be gentle on the more stressful days. That leads me to the next part of the process... practice. Practice makes progress.

Practice.

It takes time and effort to be good at taking care of oneself, especially if you were like me and had a lot more years self-deprecating than self-caring. It is one, little, concerted effort, one day at a time, and sometimes 1 hour at a time. Keep the focus on well-being and improving. Don't just *coast* and let life happen to you.

I encourage you to keep going and practice putting yourself first mentally, physically, and emotionally. Especially, when you might be hard wired to put others before your own well-being.

It takes time and practice. With time, consistency and practice, things will begin to feel more natural and you will make progress. You will start to experience those promises.

Just like zipping a zipper, things will line up and even-out, over time. Nothing needs to be forced. If you have ever tried to force a zipper to zip up, before things are lined up, you will experience resistance. No one likes resistance. When things are lined up and in order it creates a smooth process to let go and heal safely. The importance here is to trust the process and give ourselves some grace. What does that look like?

Giving Ourselves Grace.

I have yet to meet the perfect person. Many people I've met that look like they have it "all together" don't. And people that don't look like they have it all together actually tend to have a lot of peace and stability.

Like we talked about with The Beautiful Exchange, we will have to adopt healthy coping mechanisms to replace our old unhealthy ways of coping. We will have to check-in with ourselves and other people instead of our old defaults of checking-out, withdrawing and disconnecting.

Healthy coping mechanisms help build resilience and maintain emotional sobriety. This helps us stabilize. When healthy boundaries are established, then I know where I end and the other person begins.

Living with emotional sobriety puts an end to acting like "everything is okay". It gives us the opportunity to work on being well. Even in the midst of facing adversity.

This adversity may happen inside ourselves or when facing parts of our past. There are a variety of ways to find healthy outlets when problems arise. It is important to remember your personal Freedom Protocol and *add* to those healthy steps with what works for you.

Here are a few ideas: enjoying the arts, seeing live music, enjoying a show or play in person, going to a movie. How about creative expressions? Get creative with doodling, drawing on a piece of paper, heading to an arts and crafts department to get a canvas to paint on. Even if it's messy, exploring an outlet is the priority.

Reiterating a previous point made is to maintain a connection with others. Finding a support group, where you can openly share what's going on in your life, where people are not going to try to "fix" you. That is one of the most healing environments you can find for change and restoration to happen.

I get it, it can be scary at first to open up and share, but it is worth it. Hearing the stories of others can be transformative in nature as well. Especially if they are going through a similar situation.

Maybe you're coming out of a divorce? Maybe you're letting go of an old identity? Whatever you are facing, it is so important to have a daily routine, a weekly routine, and a Freedom Protocol for when triggers arise. These are the things that will prevent you from being tempted to act out and numb.

Promise to You

Your life will change as you prioritize well-being. The opposite is true if you ignore your own personal, emotional, mental and spiritual needs. You will be like the house on the side of the road that is falling apart on the outside. Most importantly on the inside.

Remember, you can't walk toward healing and toward self-sabotage at the same time. We can only walk forward or backward. Not both at the same time. So, I encourage you to walk AWAY from self-harm and TOWARD well-being. Live free. Take the way out.

Looking ahead.

Looking ahead is very important for maintaining a lifestyle of development, transformation, and deep inner healing. Part of living a fulfilling life is to set some goals and see the milestones happen on the way to those goals. This is where life begins - beyond addiction and self-destructive patterns.

Realistic goal setting and meaningful goals that align with your personal values and aspirations are very important. Seeing those goals broken into actionable steps, helps those goals become a reality.

Don't forget to celebrate progress along the way! We are all a wonderful work in progress. Throughout this process it is important to foster and nurture healthy relationships around us.

Meaningful friendships in the midst of transformation and change are very important. It takes time to develop. Quality friendships can be hard to come by. Some of the most valuable friendships to have are in the community of those who are recovering from similar pain and trauma that you have endured.

Staying in a community will help maintain long-term recovery. One of the ways to build and nurture healthy relationships is through consistency. Simply, showing up. Be where you say you're going to be, when you say you're going to be there. Acknowledge and care for the needs of others. This does take ongoing effort and it is possible. When you are ready to go to any length to be well, the opportunities are endless!

I want to encourage you to embrace a fulfilling life beyond addiction and self-sabotage and continue your journey of growth and healing. When I resigned from harming myself with bad relationships and emotional overeating, it became my full-time job to be well. This meant I had to learn from the *signals* that my body and feelings were sending.

Just like addiction and self-harm, the brain needs a bigger stronger hit to maintain that dopamine reward center. But guess what? As our brain heals, we can experience life more vividly. We can experience genuine intimacy with ourselves, God, and others. We can suck the marrow out of life, one day at a time.

As we talked about triggers in Chapter 3, we will be pricked by pain and we cannot always predict when, how or what will tempt us to backslide. The difference today is that your choice is being restored.

Today, we can implement a *Freedom Protocol* that will help us manage **when** we get triggered or tempted to act out on our **old** compulsive behavior. When we come up against a high risk situation and we don't know what to do, we can simply stop. We can pray and wait for the answer to come to us instead of reacting with whatever pops into our minds. I assure you that remaining sober in your mind, body, and relationships is available to you when you choose to work on it one day at a time.

Cravings

When cravings come we can acknowledge that they exist, but we can also acknowledge that we are prioritizing wellness. We are breaking the cycle of self-destructive patterns today.

Sometimes it's important to look at what is behind the craving. What am I trying to avoid feeling and why? Those are important to uncover. What is God wanting to heal? Is it a deep wound within you?

Maybe it is something a little like being hungry, angry, lonely or tired? Or maybe it is something deeper and more profound. When you stop harming yourself it gives an opportunity for a revelation about yourself.

That is when you find the pain you wish to trade. Ask God to come into that pain and heal it. You will keep the memory, without the pain. You can let go of sadness in exchange for peace. It is possible for you. Keep going and do not give up.

Accountability

Before we wrap up this chapter I'd like to talk about accountability. Sometimes that can feel like a "dirty word". Being accountable to someone for our actions is not always fun but it does lead to life.

Accountability is a powerful tool for personal growth and achieving goals. It involves taking responsibility for our actions, choices, and commitments. While some may perceive accountability as a negative or burdensome concept, it is important to recognize that it is not a dirty word. In fact, accountability can bring numerous benefits to our lives. Here's why:

Personal Growth: Accountability encourages self-reflection and self-awareness. When we hold ourselves accountable, we become more conscious of our behaviors, habits, and patterns. This awareness allows us to identify areas for improvement and make necessary changes, leading to personal growth and development.

Goal Achievement: Accountability plays a crucial role in goal setting and achievement. When we hold ourselves accountable, we are more likely to stay focused, motivated, and committed to our goals. It helps us track our progress, overcome obstacles, and make necessary adjustments along the way. Accountability provides the structure and discipline needed to turn aspirations into tangible results.

Building Trust and Relationships: Accountability fosters trust and strengthens relationships. When we have someone help hold us accountable, we demonstrate reliability, integrity, and a commitment to our words and actions. This builds trust with others, as they see us following through on our commitments. Accountability also encourages open communication and collaboration, as it creates a sense of responsibility and mutual respect within relationships.

Learning from Mistakes: Accountability allows us to learn from our mistakes and failures. When we take ownership of our actions, we can reflect on what went wrong, identify lessons learned, and make necessary adjustments for future success. Embracing accountability helps us grow from setbacks and turn them into valuable learning experiences.

Empowerment and Control: Accountability empowers us to take back control of our lives. It shifts the focus from external factors to our own actions and choices. By holding ourselves accountable, we recognize that we have the power to shape our circumstances and create the life we desire.

It's important to note that accountability doesn't mean being overly self-critical or punishing ourselves for mistakes. Instead, it is about taking responsibility, learning, and making positive changes. Accountability is a tool for growth, progress, and personal fortitude.

By embracing accountability, we can cultivate a mindset of self-improvement, achieve our goals, build stronger relationships, and take control of our lives. It is not a dirty word, but rather a valuable concept that can lead to positive transformation.

On the contrary, when our brains have been caught in The Addiction Cycle and self-destructive patterns have taken root in our brains, it can be hard or even impossible, to break the cycle on our own. That is why this book exists! To help bring light into when addiction strikes and regain the ability to make healthy choices, with the help of others who understand. A safe, accountability partner is key.

You have permission to ask for help. Find an accountability partner! It can be quite a challenge but it is worth it. When I prayed and waited, God brought the right person to me. I just had to be willing and open, then they were guided to me. A supernatural provision.

See what might happen if you ask and wait to see *who* might come into your life. A guide that can help hold you accountable for transformation and change. They help you stay committed to being in a place of wellness. Accountability is *like* having a Project Manager on site, to ensure the final Touches come to completion. Wholeness is yours, when you refuse to give up and participate in the process of change.

Try this:

Write down at least one part of this chapter that makes you feel a little uncomfortable. What was it? When you were reading and something stirred inside you and made you feel a little uncomfortable? Please pay attention to it. That is likely the area that needs the most tenderness and *attention* right now. Pray for the right accountability person to find their way to you and keep it simple. Let your mind stay in the day and wait for direction on the next-right-move. Just for this moment.

Chapter 8 Summary:

This is where we took note of the parallels between a building renovation project and our own transformation. This gave a realistic way evaluate our progress of inner healing, letting go, and moving forward. We looked at the importance of maintaining healthy practices, on a daily basis. We looked at practical tips for managing emotional pain, when we get triggered. We talked about protecting our wellness as a valued treasure.

Finally, we talked about the value of accountability. Accountability is NOT a dirty word. We talked about the Promises that are offered in the 12-step recovery rooms. We talked about the Beautiful Exchange. We talked about needing others. We talked about not going alone and the promise of transformation when we remain humble, honest and willing. You have permission to ask for help from God and others.

Conclusion

Wow! You did it. You courageously navigated through the waters of the demolition and reconstruction process of emotional sobriety, recovery and wellness. Wonderful job!

We looked at the problem of addiction. Wanting to stop a negative pattern, and not being able to stop when we get triggered and our brains take over. We looked at some of the underlying causes and factors that contribute to addiction and self-destructive patterns. We talked about awareness and how to stay alert to the negative impacts of the patterns from our past and the enemies of change.

We looked at the freedom protocol and the way out. We saw how the strategy for breaking negative patterns works and how to create roadblocks that will add to the solution of breaking chronic relapse and going back to old patterns. We talked about overcoming challenges and building resilience. We talked about how to stay motivated in the face of adversity. We talked about creating a supportive environment and not trying to "go it alone".

We talked about building and maintaining healthy relationships by setting boundaries and we talked about tips for finding and utilizing the rooms of recovery. We talked about walking out our healing and maintaining long-term recovery. We talked about being well.

We explored strategies for maintaining emotional sobriety and preventing relapse. We discussed the importance of self-care and prioritizing yourself over a plant, a pet, or another person. You are important.

We discussed healthy coping mechanisms that we can replace old negative destructive patterns with. We learned about creating a fulfilling life beyond addiction and self-sabotage.

Sometimes, it is okay to not be okay. To cry. It is okay to need help. Asking for help is an act of courage and humility. It is okay to admit when you feel powerless over things you cannot control, including your own brain and body. There is a way out and there is hope.

At this point it is important to take action. Don't just read the book and move on, put it into practice! If you need help we are here to help you. Visit the website and sign up for one of our workshops, private coaching or schedule your very own Freedom Protocol at GraceRevealedLLC.com/book.

Final Words of Encouragement

I leave you with hope to keep going no matter what. Your life matters. When you are well, you will help heal others. Please don't give up. Remember, "Hurt people, hurt people"?

Well, guess what? "Healed people, heal people". I repeat: Healed people, heal people. Let that sink in.

If you found this to be helpful, please share it with a friend, family member or loved one. Pass it on to someone who desperately wants change. If you are in a dark season, please remember that "this too shall pass". There is hope and there is healing available to you. It happens faster, when you *prioritize* well-being. Also, stay connected. Visit my social media channels at the end of this book. Look forward to meeting you and hearing about your transformation. At any point you feel stuck, schedule a free call with us. No need to try going it alone anymore. You've come so far!

Change is not easy but it is good. It is not for the weak but for the courageous. The courageous will tap into a life worth living! Live! Happy, joyous and free from the chains that once bound you.

May love, courage, willingness, and the desire to change come to you at the right place at the right time. Be the miracle. Walk out the amazing life that you know you were meant to live. One day, or simply just one moment at a time.

The End.

..Or is it just the beginning?

Grace Revealed LLC

Layla Grace, is Myrtle Beach area Chamber of Commerce winner of the 2020 Entrepreneur of the Year award. Layla is recognized for innovative ways to help businesses manage stress and avoid burnout.

Layla went from debilitating burnout, adrenal fatigue, chronic stress, and self-destructive patterns, to - enjoying life, stability, and peace of mind. Does that resonate with you?

Battling stress alone is dangerous. She is living proof of a life transformed and has dedicated her time to helping others avoid toxic stress that causes burnout and chronic relapse. Understanding how unmanaged stress can progress, Grace Revealed makes the burnout prevention process simple. Offering the Freedom Protocol gives users a way out of the addiction cycle.

Layla helps reveal the roots of stress, anxiety, and burnout so you can change the fruit. She empowers you to effectively turn yourself and your team around in a lively, practical way. When you are struggling or simply wanting practical tools to enhance your life, Layla will guide you to well-being. See upcoming events or invite her to speak at one of your events at GraceRevealedLLC.com to stay connected.

Stay In Touch

Fun Freebies
Sign Up for Layla's Weekly Wellness emails here: www.GraceRevealedLLC.com

Social Media
Follow Layla on Instagram: @laylagracer

Subscribe to Layla's YouTube channel:
https://www.instagram.com/gracerevealedllc

https://www.facebook.com/Graceful1s/

https://www.youtube.com/@GraceRevealed

https://www.linkedin.com/company/grace-revealed-llc

https://www.linkedin.com/in/layla-grace-1607b164/

Subscribe to Jayla In the Morning - Josh & Layla's Marriage Tips:
https://www.youtube.com/@JaylaIntheMorning
https://www.instagram.com/jaylainthemornings

ACKNOWLEDGEMENTS

To my dear loving husband, Joshua Michael Alan Rule. You truly are the most well rounded human being I've ever met. Faithful and True. My "steady wind". Where would I be without you?

Thank you for all your time and dedication to help this book become a reality. You truly are my No Matter What.

To Roger and Shirley Coons, my Spiritual Father and Mother

You are more than just The Blessing, but a true example of Love In Action. Thank you for believing in me and being The Best cheerleaders I've ever met.

A special thanks to the work of Marnie C. Ferree at Bethesda Workshops in Nashville, TN.

Marnie's timeless work in her book *No Stones* helped to anchor my transformation. My time in the 2018 Healing for Women workshop saved my life. I am forever grateful for your courage and commitment to be well.

Finally, a special thanks to courageous men and women in the 12-Step rooms of Recovery that fight to be well, one day at a time. You carry the message.

Layla Grace is the Director of Grace Revealed, LLC and a renowned Burnout Prevention specialist. With a passion for helping individuals overcome self-destructive patterns, Layla has dedicated her life to guiding others towards emotional sobriety and a path of healing. Recipient of the prestigious 2020 Entrepreneur of the Year Award from the Myrtle Beach area Chamber of Commerce, Layla has been recognized for her exceptional contributions in the field of personal development. Drawing from her own experiences as a survivor of childhood and adult trauma, she has emerged as a beacon of hope and resilience. As a sought-after public speaker, Layla has captivated audiences around the world with her powerful message of overcoming shame and breaking the cycle of chronic relapse. Her personal journey of recovery from addiction, which began in March of 2018, serves as a testament to the transformative power of perseverance and self-discovery. In her groundbreaking book, "Relapse No More: The Way Out," Layla shares invaluable insights and practical strategies for achieving emotional sobriety. With a compassionate and empathetic approach, she provides readers with the tools they need to navigate the challenges of self-destructive patterns and find lasting healing.

Visit: **www.GraceRevealedLLC.com** today to learn more about inviting Layla Grace to speak at your upcoming event or attend a Grace Revealed Wellness workshop.

Send inquiries, testimonials and positive remarks to: info@gracerevealedllc.com

Printed in the USA
CPSIA information can be obtained
at www.ICGtesting.com
JSHW070511260124
55837JS00003B/3

9 798218 338473